Also Available From the American Academy of Pediatrics

Common Conditions

ADHD: What Every Parent Needs to Know

Allergies and Asthma: What Every Parent Needs to Know

The Big Book of Symptoms: A–Z Guide to Your Child's Health

Mama Doc Medicine: Finding Calm and Confidence in Parenting, Child Health, and Work-Life Balance

My Child Is Sick! Expert Advice for Managing Common Illnesses and Injuries

Sleep: What Every Parent Needs to Know

Developmental, Behavioral, and Psychosocial Information

Autism Spectrum Disorders: What Every Parent Needs to Know

Building Resilience in Children and Teens: Giving Kids Roots and Wings

CyberSafe: Protecting and Empowering Kids in the Digital World of Texting, Gaming, and Social Media

Mental Health, Naturally: The Family Guide to Holistic Care for a Healthy Mind and Body

Raising Kids to Thrive: Balancing Love With Expectations and Protection With Trust

Newborns, Infants, and Toddlers

Caring for Your Baby and Young Child: Birth to Age 5*

Dad to Dad: Parenting Like a Pro

Guide to Toilet Training*

Heading Home With Your Newborn: From Birth to Reality

Mommy Calls: Dr. Tanya Answers Parents' Top 101 Questions About Babies and Toddlers

New Mother's Guide to Breastfeeding*

Newborn Intensive Care: What Every Parent Needs to Know

Raising Twins: Parenting Multiples From Pregnancy Through the School Years

Retro Baby: Cut Back on All the Gear and Boost Your Baby's Development With More Than 100 Time-Tested Activities

Your Baby's First Year*

Nutrition and Fitness

Food Fights: Winning the Nutritional Challenges of Parenthood Armed With Insight, Humor, and a Bottle of Ketchup

Nutrition: What Every Parent Needs to Know

A Parent's Guide to Childhood Obesity: A Road Map to Health

Sports Success R_x! Your Child's Prescription for the Best Experience

School-aged Children and Adolescents

Less Stress, More Success: A New Approach to Guiding Your Teen Through College Admissions and Beyond

For additional parenting resources, visit the HealthyChildren bookstore at **shop.aap.org/for-parents**.

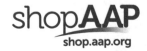

shop.aap.org

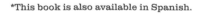

W9-BZU-746

For more information on bedwetting and Dr Bennett's other books, please visit his website, www.howardjbennett.com.

Waking Up Dry

A GUIDE TO HELP CHILDREN OVERCOME BEDWETTING

2nd Edition

HOWARD J. BENNETT, MD, FAAP

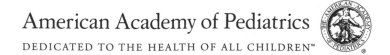

American Academy of Pediatrics
DEDICATED TO THE HEALTH OF ALL CHILDREN™

American Academy of Pediatrics Publishing Staff

Director, Department of Publishing
Mark Grimes

Director, Division of Professional and
Consumer Publishing
Jeff Mahony

Manager, Consumer Publishing
Kathryn Sparks

Coordinator, Product Development
Holly Kaminski

Director, Division of Editorial and Production
Services
Sandi King, MS

Editorial Specialist
Amanda Cozza

Publishing and Production Services
Specialist
Shannan Martin

Manager, Art Direction and Production
Peg Mulcahy

Director, Department of Marketing and Sales
Mary Lou White

Manager, Consumer Product Marketing
Mary Jo Reynolds

About the American Academy of Pediatrics

The American Academy of Pediatrics is an organization of 62,000 primary care pediatricians, pediatric medical subspecialists, and pediatric surgical specialists dedicated to the health, safety, and well-being of infants, children, adolescents, and young adults.

Published by the American Academy of Pediatrics
141 Northwest Point Blvd, Elk Grove Village, IL 60007-1019
847/434-4000
Fax: 847/434-8000
www.aap.org

Cover photography by Patricia Mathes Lake
Original artwork in publication by John Regnier and Peg Mulcahy

Second Edition—2015
First Edition—2005

Library of Congress Control Number: 2014935004
ISBN: 978-1-58110-906-1
eBook: 978-1-58110-907-8
EPUB: 978-1-58110-908-5
Kindle: 978-1-58110-909-2

The recommendations in this publication do not indicate an exclusive course of treatment or serve as a standard of medical care. Variations, taking into account individual circumstances, may be appropriate.

Statements and opinions expressed are those of the authors and not necessarily those of the American Academy of Pediatrics.

The American Academy of Pediatrics does not review or endorse any modifications made to this document and in no event shall the American Academy of Pediatrics be liable for any such changes.

Products and Web sites are mentioned for informational purposes only. Inclusion in this publication does not imply an endorsement by the American Academy of Pediatrics. The American Academy of Pediatrics is not responsible for the content of the resources mentioned in this publication. Web site addresses are as current as possible but may change at any time.

The persons whose photographs are depicted in this publication are professional models. They have no relation to the issues discussed. Any characters they are portraying are fictional.

Every effort has been made to keep *Waking Up Dry: A Guide to Help Children Overcome Bedwetting* consistent with the most recent advice and information available from the American Academy of Pediatrics.

This book has been developed by the American Academy of Pediatrics. The authors, editors, and contributors are expert authorities in the field of pediatrics. No commercial involvement of any kind has been solicited or accepted in the development of the content of this publication.

Special discounts are available for bulk purchases of this book. E-mail our Special Sales Department at aapsales@aap.org for more information.

CB0087
9-361 /0315   1 2 3 4 5 6 7 8 9 10

What People Are Saying

I recommend *Waking Up Dry* to every family I see with a bed-wetter. Dr Bennett knows more about this symptom than anyone else in pediatrics or urology. Overcoming bedwetting takes motivation, endurance, and self-study. This book is the answer. It covers every imaginable parent question, and the advice is evidence- and experience-based.

Barton Schmitt, MD, FAAP
Professor of Pediatrics, University of Colorado School of Medicine
Director, Enuresis-Encopresis Clinic, Children's Hospital Colorado

Dr Bennett's child-friendly and humorous style comes through loud and clear in the pages of this superb and recently updated book on overcoming bedwetting....I highly recommend this as the #1 practical resource book for children, parents, and health care professionals. It's the best I've seen yet.

Lawrence A. Vitulano, PhD
Associate Clinical Professor of Psychology
Child Study Center
Yale University

Bennett's superb book outlining issues regarding bedwetting is an excellent guide for understanding what bedwetting is and how to best approach managing the problem. Complete, well written, clever in its design, and very parent and child friendly, this book is a valuable addition to the parents' library of well-established references for helping them raise their children compassionately, knowledgeably, and with well-placed confidence. Outstanding approach from an experienced pediatrician.

Steven P. Shelov, MD, MS, FAAP
Associate Dean, Undergraduate Medical Education,
    Winthrop University Hospital, Clinical Regional Campus
Professor of Pediatrics, Stony Brook School of Medicine

For my patients, who taught me about
bedwetting as I developed this program.

Contents

BE SURE TO READ THIS PART OF THE BOOK!

Contents

Acknowledgments

Although this book is a written account of my Waking Up Dry Program, a number of people helped it grow from a clinical protocol to an actual book. First, I would like to thank Monica Adler for suggesting I "take my show on the road." Without her enthusiasm and good-natured prodding, this book would never have been written. I would also like to thank the following friends and colleagues who reviewed the manuscript: Linda Goldstein, MD, FAAP; Inas Anderson, MD, FAAP; Barry Belman, MD, FAAP; Dale Gertz, MD, FAAP; William Hulbert, MD, FAAP; and Mandy Katz. Debbie Gilbert, MLS, AHIP, was instrumental in helping me track down references I needed to review. I got some additional help from William S. Haubrich, MD, and Angie Cheek, VMD, who provided information I needed for some of the filler I used in the book. I would also like to thank my wife, Jan, who not only picked up the slack whenever I disappeared into the basement to work on the book, but also provided terrific insight when she read the manuscript in its earliest stages.

Because no one practices medicine in a vacuum, I would like to thank my clinical teachers and all of the people who have conducted research on bedwetting. In particular, I would like to thank Barton Schmitt, MD, FAAP, whose writings on bedwetting have had a big influence on how I approach the condition.

I am very grateful for everyone at the American Academy of Pediatrics who helped make this project a reality. Eileen Glasstetter and Mark Grimes saw the potential in a self-help book that spoke directly to children. Amanda Cozza is a copy editor extraordinaire, and Peg Mulcahy did a terrific job giving the book an appealing look that children will appreciate. Holly Kaminski did a great job pulling everything together so children will have a book they can really use.

Introduction for Kids

Your parents bought this book because they want to help you become dry at night. I'm a pediatrician (a kid's doctor), and I've been helping children overcome bedwetting for more than 30 years. This book describes the program I use with patients in my office. I wrote the book because my Waking Up Dry Program really works, and a number of parents and doctor friends encouraged me to write about what I do.

Bedwetting is not a serious medical condition, but it can be very difficult to live with. Wetting at night makes it hard to go on sleepovers, it makes you feel uncomfortable in the morning, and worst of all, it's upsetting not to have control over your body while you sleep. But the good news is you can do something about it. With motivation and practice, you can become the boss of your body! (Motivation means you want something bad enough to work hard for it.)

If you tried to stop bedwetting in the past and it didn't work, I can understand you might not want to try something new. The main reason programs fail is because children don't get enough support to make it through the rough spots. The Waking Up Dry Program has a winning record for many reasons. First, it includes lots of tips that help you along the way. Second, the program attacks the problem from different angles. Third, and most important, it lets you play a big role in setting up and carrying out the program.

When I work with children in my office, I talk to them as much as I talk to their parents. In the same way, I will be talking directly to you throughout the book. I will also be giving your parents special instructions along the way because we need their help to make the program work. In my office, I tell kids that I will be their coach and their parents will be my assistant coaches. You are the player! You are the star! You will also be the one who does most of the work. One of the things I will say over and over is how important it is for you to be involved with the program. Whether it's filling out your Waking Up Dry calendar or following the steps of the program with your coaches, the more motivated you are, the more likely you will become dry. I wrote this book for children of different ages, so if you are a younger reader, you may need your *coach* (mom or dad) to read the book to you. That's OK. That's one of the things coaches do. In fact, your coach needs to read the book with you even if she doesn't need to read it to you. Some of the information in the book can be complicated, even for good readers, and going through it with your coaches will improve your chances of becoming dry. Also, your coaches need to help out with many parts of the program, so reading the book together can be really fun. Together, all of us will work hard so you can start waking up every morning in a nice dry bed.

Finally, I want you to know that I love being a pediatrician, and one of my greatest joys as a doctor is helping kids become dry at night. So even though I won't become your personal doctor, I hope my book will help you beat bedwetting forever!

Dr B

Introduction for Parents

It's been known for a long time that bedwetting resolves on its own in most cases. Every year, 15% of children who wet the bed become dry without any intervention. This fact has led many doctors to simply reassure patients that the condition is not serious and will go away on its own. The problem with this approach is that bedwetting can affect a child's self-esteem. Therefore, it's shortsighted to ask a child to wait years to become dry if treatment can expedite the process. On the other hand, given the rate of spontaneous improvement, you should always consider the following things before starting any treatment: Is your child motivated to become dry? Is the treatment safe?

Some doctors prescribe medication to stop bedwetting. Although medication may be helpful, it doesn't cure the problem, and one of the drugs used to treat bedwetting (imipramine) has potentially serious side effects. Many doctors appropriately inform parents about behavior management techniques (including a special device called the bedwetting alarm), which are the most effective treatments for bedwetting. Unfortunately, exploring the many facets of treatment is difficult to accomplish during routine checkups, and doctors often don't have the time needed to do this. For example, although bedwetting alarms come with instructions, a child's chances of becoming dry increase dramatically if an experienced practitioner helps her avoid the pitfalls associated with treatment. The information in this book is designed to provide that guidance. There are a few things you should know right away.

- While much of the book is directed toward children, you are an essential part of the program. (Even highly motivated children need their parents' assistance to make the program work.)

- Bedwetting is not your fault. You will learn more about the causes of bedwetting in Chapter 3, but for now, let go of any guilt you've been carrying around for the past few years.
- Bedwetting is not your child's fault either. No one wets the bed on purpose. However, because bedwetting can be draining both physically and emotionally, parents may feel a sense of frustration, helplessness, and anger when they have to deal with wet beds day after day.
- It's important that you present a positive attitude to your child throughout the program because negative emotions undermine what we're trying to accomplish. (Even subtle signs of disapproval can result in more wetting.) Think of yourself as a soccer coach who always says something uplifting, even when a player stumbles and misses the ball: "Great effort, Alex. I know you'll stop the ball next time!"
- It's equally important that you and your child are prepared and motivated to do the program. Teaching children to be dry means extra laundry, having to coax and support them when they're frustrated, and negotiating with your spouse over who's helping with which part of the program. For the child, it means using the bedwetting alarm and having to deal with fatigue because the alarm wakes you up at night. But by working together, you can overcome these obstacles and end up with a child who is dry at night.
- Despite these challenges, helping your child become dry can be one of the most gratifying experiences you will have as a parent!

In Chapter 6, I give children an assignment to find out how motivated they are to become dry at night. Right now, I'd like to be more philosophical about the issue of readiness. Consciously or otherwise, society puts pressure on parents for their children to achieve developmental goals at specific times. Most of us have worried about our children because they were a little late with one skill or another. Because evaluating a child's development is a big part of general pediatrics, I spend a lot of time reassuring parents that their children are normal and recommending that we give them time to develop at their own pace.

T. Berry Brazelton, MD, FAAP, was one of the first pediatricians to call for a child-oriented approach to toilet training and bladder control, and those same principles should be applied to the Waking Up Dry Program. Dr Brazelton told parents 50 years ago to hold off on potty training until the child showed signs that she was ready. If parents waited for these cues, toileting usually proceeded smoothly. If they didn't, the process was prolonged or they ran into difficulty.

Although there is no magic age when children are ready to work on their wetting, most children show some awareness of the problem by the time they are 5 to 6 years old. (This is the age when children realize their friends are no longer wearing Pull-Ups to bed.) Whether or not children say anything about this depends on their personalities and how they approach learning new skills. Some children communicate their worries directly. Others keep things to themselves or, surprisingly, overcompensate by acting out. If your child has said something to you about wanting to be dry, it's appropriate to use the book. If your child is oblivious about her wetting, you can read the book yourself so you're prepared to deal with the situation once she becomes ready. (There is a lot of practical advice in the book, which will make living with bedwetting easier.) If you sense that your child wants to be dry, but she hasn't said anything about it, you can explore this area to see if your hunch is correct. The best time to talk with your child is when she is well rested, well fed, and free of distractions. If your child responds positively to these queries, you can use the book. If she doesn't, put it away for a while, but keep your radar turned on for signs that she has changed her mind. Here are some ways to find out if your child is interested in becoming dry.

- Ask your child if there is anything about being wet (or wearing Pull-Ups) that she doesn't like.
- Ask your child if she would like to stop wearing Pull-Ups.
- Ask your child if she would like to be dry at night.
- If you or a relative wet the bed as kids, share this information with your child so she knows someone else in the family had the same problem she does. You can help children talk about their feelings if you go first: "When I was your age, I hated waking up in a wet bed."
- Tell your child you bought a book that teaches kids how to be dry at night. Let her know the book is fun to read and will show her how to be the boss of her body.

Finally, please note that the book is not meant to treat children with complicated forms of bedwetting. While most children with nighttime wetting do not have a medical condition that underlies the problem, it's important to exclude such possibilities before you start the program (see Chapter 4).

Howard J. Bennett

How to Use This Book

It's normal for kids to want to jump into the program right after they get the book. Although I know you're eager to start, it's important to read the book from the beginning. The reason for this is that some of the things at the end of the book build on information I discuss earlier. There are a few chapters, however, that you may want to look at right away: Sleepovers (Chapter 22) and What to Do if Someone Discovers Your Supplies (Chapter 23).

I spent a lot of time thinking about ways to make the book easier to use. One of the ideas I had come up with was to highlight certain sections within each chapter.

The following guides describe the special sections you will see in the book:

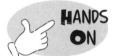 **HANDS ON** A Hands On box refers to activities you can do to better understand the way your body works.

 KID'S ALERT A Kid's Alert box refers to parts of the program you should pay close attention to.

FUN FACTS When I researched the book, I had found a lot of cool facts that I wanted to share with you and your coaches. Although some of them are not directly related to the program, I think you'll both enjoy them. Each one is in its own Fun Facts box.

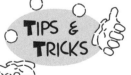 **TIPS & TRICKS** There are lots of practical ideas in the book. The Tips & Tricks box refers to certain ones I wanted to bring to your attention.

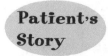

Patient's Story

As you read the book, you will find some stories from actual patients of mine. I included these stories to highlight certain points. These are all real people and real stories, but the names are made up. Each one is in its own Patient's Story box.

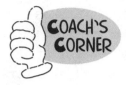

COACH'S CORNER

The Coach's Corner box refers to a section at the back of most chapters that's specifically for your coaches.

Because I want to help as many children as possible, I wrote the book so you can do the program at home with your parents. Don't forget, however, that your doctor is also interested in helping you become dry. There are a few advantages to working with a medical professional: we've done this before, and we can sometimes motivate kids better than parents. If you use the book with your doctor, he or she may change the program a little. That's OK because we each have our own way of doing things.

Here is a summary of the information you will find in the book.

- **Part 1** describes how many kids wet the bed, how your body works, and why kids are wet at night. It contains a questionnaire to help you figure out the type of wetting you have.
- **Part 2** tests your motivation for becoming dry by having you do the same dry-bed homework I give patients in my office. This consists of 4 tasks: going to the bathroom when you need to, making a calendar to keep track of your wet and dry nights, finding out the size of your bladder, and determining if you can wake up at night to loud sound.
- **Part 3** shows you how to score your dry-bed homework and introduces you to some bladder exercises and other parts of the program.
- **Part 4** describes the bedwetting alarm, which is the most successful tool you can use to become dry at night.

- **Part 5** shows you how to set up the Waking Up Dry Program. It includes a contract that you and your coaches will sign.
- **Part 6** includes chapters on sleepovers, what to do if someone finds your bedwetting supplies, and other techniques that can help you stay dry at night.
- **Part 7** is for coaches. It includes lots of tips to help you make it through the rough spots, tips on dealing with wet beds, and information on medicine that some kids need to become dry.

The appendixes include additional information for you, your coaches, and your doctor. You can download some sections from the appendix by visiting the book page of my website: www.howardjbennett.com.

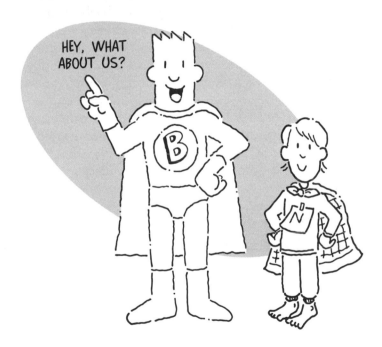

Oh, I almost forgot. Throughout the book, you will notice a couple of characters hanging around making helpful or silly comments. Bladderman is the one in the official costume, and

Nick is the one in regular clothes. Bladderman graduated from superhero school years ago. Nick wants to be a superhero when he grows up, but right now he's working with Bladderman to become dry at night.

COACH'S CORNER

Research has shown that children are more motivated to become dry if they are actively involved with the treatment plan. This gives kids a sense of ownership for the program and increases their chances for success. Although *Waking Up Dry* is a parenting book, I want children to see it as *their* book as well.

To help accomplish this goal, I organized the book so I am talking to them the same way I do with patients in my office. Given the age range of children who wet at night, this proved to be a bit of a challenge. While I did not want to talk down to older kids, I also did not want to overload or confuse younger ones. To make this work, I need your help. **If you come across material that looks too complicated for your child, edit or condense what you read to make it easier.** This will not only keep your child interested in the book but it will help him do a better job understanding the program.

Although becoming dry is everyone's ultimate goal, children have lots of small successes (as well as setbacks) before they complete the program. It's important to praise your child when you notice these gains because it lets him know you're proud of his accomplishments. (It also motivates him to work on the program.)

Look for success in the following areas:
- Enthusiasm about the book
- Asking questions about his body or the program
- Cooperation with the program

- Showing responsibility for doing a task
- Carrying out a task properly
- Making gains with any part of the program (eg, filling out his calendar, doing his bladder exercises)
- Waking up to the bedwetting alarm
- Having smaller wet spots or wetting later in the night
- Having fewer wet episodes per night
- Waking up on his own to pee
- Having dry nights

While there is no set age when children are ready to work on becoming dry, most of the kids I treat are 6 years and older. (Bedwetting is so common that most doctors don't consider it to be a health problem until children are 6 years old.) As you read through the book, you may find that your child will do better with a low-key approach. This means you can skip the dry-bed homework and stick with the easier aspects of the program (see Katie's Story on page 47). In addition, Chapter 28 summarizes which parts of the program are appropriate for children according to their ages.

PART 1

Facts About Bedwetting

CHAPTER 1

You Are Not Alone

Michael's Story

Michael is a 9-year-old boy who saw me for a bedwetting visit a few years ago. When I entered the room, Michael was sitting on a chair next to his mom and dad. His arms were folded in his lap, and his face was pointed toward the floor.

I knew right away that Michael was embarrassed about coming to see me. I started the visit by asking him lots of questions about school and his favorite hobbies. After a few minutes, Michael brightened up and we started talking about why kids wet at night and what they can do to become dry. When I told Michael how many children wet the bed, his jaw dropped. He couldn't believe it. All these years he thought he was the only one who woke up every morning in a cold, wet bed. As I watched Michael's face, I saw a huge burden melt away like a snowman on a warm afternoon. The rest of the visit sailed by. Michael became dry 4 weeks after he started the program.

One of the first things I tell kids at bedwetting visits is they are not the only ones who have trouble staying dry at night. Because bedwetting is a private matter, people usually do not talk about it outside the family. As a result, most children (and some parents) think they are the only ones who have the problem. This is not true. Although it's hard to believe, there are more

than 5 million children in the United States who wet the bed.
I will discuss why this happens in Chapter 3. Right now, I want
to give you a sense of how big the number 5 *million* really is.

- If 5 million elephants were lined up end to end, they would
  stretch all the way around the world.
- If you built a tower out of 5 million soccer balls, it would be
  taller than the Washington Monument.
- If you invited 5 million children to see a professional baseball
  game, you would need 100 stadiums to find them all seats.

When I see children at work, they often ask me how many
kids their own age wet the bed. The best way to understand
these numbers is to figure out how many kids wet the bed in different
grades at school. First, we'll look at children in elementary
school. Let's say we take a school that has 500 children from
kindergarten to fifth grade (this means the school has kids
ranging from 5 to 10 years of age). Table 1-1 shows how many
kids wet the bed in each grade.

When you add up these numbers, it turns out that in an elementary
school of 500 children, 50 are wet at night!

Table 1-1.
Number of Students Who Wet the Bed in an Elementary School of 500 Children

Grade	Number Who Wet the Bed
Fifth	🧍🧍🧍🧍 (4)
Fourth	🧍🧍🧍🧍🧍 (5)
Third	🧍🧍🧍🧍🧍🧍 (6)
Second	🧍🧍🧍🧍🧍🧍🧍🧍 (8)
First	🧍🧍🧍🧍🧍🧍🧍🧍🧍🧍 (10)
Kindergarten	🧍🧍🧍🧍🧍🧍🧍🧍🧍🧍🧍🧍🧍🧍🧍🧍🧍 (17)

Krista's Story

A few years ago, I saw a 10-year-old girl for a bedwetting visit. When I told Krista how many kids are wet at night, she did not look relieved. Instead, she focused on the fifth-grade numbers: "You mean there are only 4 kids in my grade who wet the bed?" I told her that was actually a large number, but sensing her disappointment I did some homework. I found out there are approximately 50,000 elementary schools in the United States. If there are 4 fifth graders at each school who wet the bed that means there are 200,000 fifth graders in the country with the same problem. That number made Krista feel a lot better.

Now let's do the same thing for middle school. Because middle schools are usually bigger than elementary schools, we'll take a school that has 1,000 children from sixth through eighth grade (this means the school has kids ranging from 11 to 13 years of age). Table 1-2 shows how many kids wet the bed in each grade.

When you add up these numbers, it turns out that in a middle school of 1,000 children, 31 are wet at night!

Now comes the interesting part. When you add up the thousands and thousands of schools in our country, you can see why there are more than 5 million children in the United States who wet the bed at night. *YOU ARE NOT ALONE!*

Table 1-2.
Number of Students Who Wet the Bed in a Middle School of 1,000 Children

Grade	Number Who Wet the Bed
Eighth	🚶🚶🚶🚶🚶🚶🚶🚶 (8)
Seventh	🚶🚶🚶🚶🚶🚶🚶🚶🚶🚶 (10)
Sixth	🚶🚶🚶🚶🚶🚶🚶🚶🚶🚶🚶🚶🚶 (13)

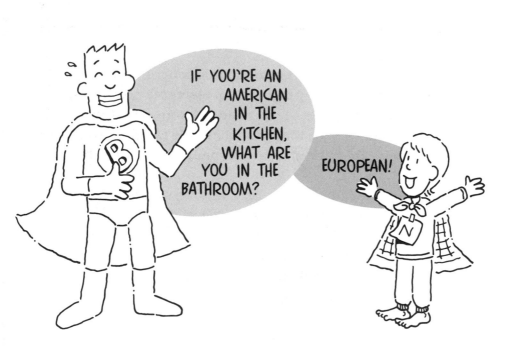

IF YOU'RE AN AMERICAN IN THE KITCHEN, WHAT ARE YOU IN THE BATHROOM?

EUROPEAN!

COACH'S CORNER

My son had his 6-year-old checkup 2 months ago. I wanted to discuss his bedwetting, but I was unsure about bringing it up with the doctor.

Every day, millions of American children wake up not knowing if their bed will be wet or dry. Bedwetting is almost as common as asthma, but it is often not discussed, even with doctors, because of its embarrassing nature.

According to a recent study, there is a communication breakdown between parents and doctors on this issue. While 82% of parents want health care professionals to discuss bedwetting, most feel uncomfortable initiating the discussion themselves. Furthermore, 68% of parents said their children's doctor has never asked about bedwetting at routine checkups.

So why aren't parents and doctors talking to each other about bedwetting? Parents are either embarrassed about the problem or assume the doctor can't help them. Doctors assume parents would ask about bedwetting if it were a concern. The prescription for this is simple. Doctors need to ask about bedwetting at routine checkups, and parents need to be more proactive by asking for help if they have a child who is wet at night.

My husband wet the bed until he was 7, but my 9-year-old is still wet at night. When will he become dry?

Every year, 15% of children become dry on their own. Although children usually follow the same pattern as their parents, this is not always the case. Because there is no way to predict when your son will overcome his wetting, I recommend you start the program if he's motivated to become dry.

continued on next page

Is it true that boys wet the bed more than girls?

Before adolescence, boys wet the bed twice as often as girls. After puberty, the numbers equal out.

My daughter used to wet the bed every night, but now she's dry half the time. What percentage of 11-year-olds are still wet at night?

I always use the school-based statistics with children because those numbers are easier to understand. Table 1-3 illustrates how many children wet the bed at different ages.

Is there a difference between children who wet the bed once a week versus 6 times a week?

As you'll learn in Chapter 4, the medical term for bedwetting is *nocturnal enuresis*. It's difficult to get good data on the incidence of enuresis because authors use different criteria to define the condition. Some diagnose enuresis if a child wets 1 or more times per month. Others diagnose the condition if a child wets 2 or more times per week. The statistics in Table 1-3 come from numerous sources that use both criteria.

A recent study involving 14,000 British children found a big difference if you looked at children who wet less than twice a week versus 2 or more times per week. As you'd expect, more children wet the bed once or twice a week than every night. Frequent bedwetters are also less likely to become dry on their own.

A study from 1996 looked at the frequency of bedwetting. The authors found that children were just as likely to have psychological problems associated with bedwetting whether they wet the bed 4 times a month or 4 times a week. This means adults should pay attention to a child's concerns about bedwetting regardless of how often it happens.

Table 1-3.
Percentage of Children Who Wet the Bed According to Age

Age (years)	Percent Who Are Wet (%)
5-year-olds	20%
6-year-olds	12%
7-year-olds	10%
8-year-olds	7%
9-year-olds	6%
10-year-olds	5%
11-year-olds	4%
12-year-olds	3%
13-year-olds	2.5%
14-year-olds	2%
15-year-olds	1.5%
16-year-olds	1%

CHAPTER 2

How Your Body Works

The title of this chapter is a little misleading. If I taught you how your entire body works, it would take hundreds of pages. Also, because this is a book about becoming dry at night, it wouldn't help much if I discussed how you breathe or why your poop smells bad. So I'll concentrate on something called the *urinary tract* (see Figure 2-1).

The urinary tract is the part of the body that makes urine, stores urine, and tells you when it's time to find a bathroom—or a tree if you're in the woods. (*Urine* is the grown-up word for pee.)

**Figure 2-1.
Urinary Tract**

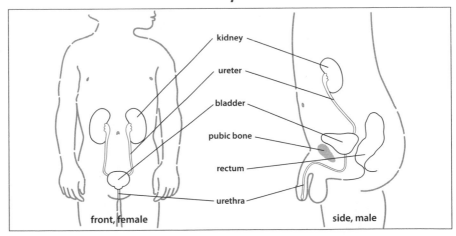

Why Do People Make Urine?

Our bodies are made up of billions of tiny parts called *cells*.
We have many different kinds of cells in our bodies—muscle
cells, brain cells, and skin cells, to name a few. Each cell has a
job. Muscle cells help us move; brain cells help us think; and
skin cells protect us from germs and other things that can hurt
our bodies. Each cell is like a tiny machine, and our cells need
energy to work, just like a car needs gasoline to run. We get
this energy from the food we eat, which is why your parents
are always bugging you to eat well.

Our cells produce waste that the body must get rid of to keep
us healthy. One of the systems the body uses to accomplish this
task is the urinary tract. Some of the waste our cells make goes
into our blood. The blood is then filtered through our *kidneys*,
which make urine.

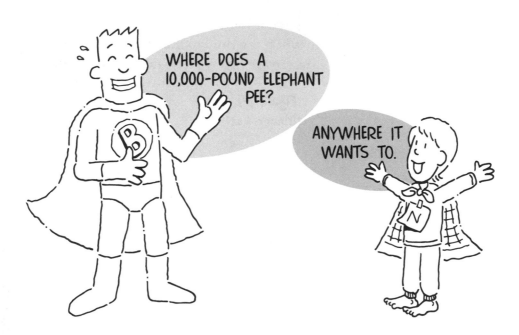

How Do the Kidneys Make Urine?

The kidneys are like special filters that remove waste and extra water from the blood. Each kidney has about 1 million tiny filters called *nephrons* (NEF-rons) that do this important work. To remove these waste products, all of the blood in your body passes through your kidneys hundreds of times per day. As the blood passes through each nephron, a tiny amount of urine is made. These tiny drops of urine then pass to a collecting area before draining out of the kidney.

FUN FACT Your body works hard to keep you healthy, even while you're sleeping. During sleep, your heart is beating, your lungs are breathing, your intestines are digesting the food you ate for dinner, and your kidneys are filtering your blood to make urine.

Where Are the Kidneys Located?

Your kidneys are located below your rib cage on each side of your body (you can't feel them because they're way in the back, behind your intestines). Because kidneys are located in the middle of our bodies, we need a way for the urine to get out. Fortunately, our body has an answer for this problem, and it's called the *bladder.*

What Is the Bladder?

The bladder is a muscular pouch (like a balloon made of muscle) that stores urine. It's located about 4 inches below your belly button and is shaped a little like an upside-down triangle. You can find your bladder by putting your hands on your body just above your penis or vagina (no giggling!). If you push down, you will feel something hard under your fingers. This is your pubic bone. The bladder is right behind the pubic bone.

How Does the Bladder Work?

After the kidneys make urine, it trickles down to the bladder through 2 tubes called the *ureters* (YUR-ah-ters). As your bladder fills up with urine, it sends a signal to your brain letting you know it's time to pee. If you're near a bathroom when this happens, you simply go to the toilet and pee. If you can't get to a bathroom right away, you try to hold it for a while. There are a few things people do to hold back urine. First, if the urge to pee is mild, your brain tells your bladder to "cool it" and the bladder relaxes so it can hold more urine. Second, if your bladder is too full to relax, you squeeze a special muscle to hold in your urine until you can get to a bathroom. This is called the *sphincter* (sss-FINK-ter) *muscle* (see Figure 2-2). There's an experiment on page 15 that demonstrates how your bladder fills up with urine the same way a balloon fills up with water.

Figure 2-2.
Urinary Tract With Sphincter Muscle

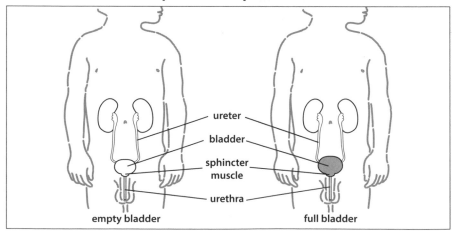

ureter

bladder

sphincter muscle

urethra

empty bladder   full bladder

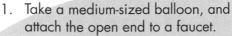

HANDS ON

1. Take a medium-sized balloon, and attach the open end to a faucet.
2. Turn on the faucet, and slowly fill the balloon with water until it's the size of a large orange.
3. Remove the balloon from the faucet, being careful to not spray water all over yourself or your coach.
4. Squeeze the neck of the balloon with your thumb and index finger, and turn the balloon upside down. (The neck of the balloon is the thin part that's right behind the opening.)
5. The balloon now looks something like your bladder.
6. Hold the balloon over the sink, and relax your thumb and index finger slightly. Water will flow from the opening the same way it comes out of your bladder when you pee.
7. Squeeze the balloon's neck, and notice that the water stops coming out. This is the same way your sphincter muscle works. If you squeeze your sphincter muscle while you're peeing, it will stop the stream and keep the rest of the urine in your bladder. If you squeeze your sphincter muscle when your bladder is full, the urine will stay inside.

SQUEEZING YOUR SPHINCTER MUSCLE FEELS THE SAME AS SQUEEZING YOUR "BOTTOM" MUSCLES WHEN YOU'RE TRYING TO HOLD IN A POOP.

Some children have trouble understanding how their bladders can send a signal to their brains telling them it's time to pee. Most kids realize they feel a tickle or pressure sensation when they need to go, but the "signal thing" confuses them. The reason the bladder is able to do this is because we have something in our bodies called *nerves*. Nerves are special cells that work like tiny telephone wires sending information from one part of the body to another. Try the experiment below and you'll see what I'm talking about.

HANDS ON Sit on a chair and have one of your coaches stand in front of you. Place your hands on your legs and close your eyes. Have your coach gently touch one of your hands. Can you tell which hand is being touched? How can you do that if your eyes are closed? The answer is you felt it. When your coach touches your hand, the feeling nerves in your skin send a signal to your brain telling you that you've been touched. If you didn't have nerves in your skin, you wouldn't know you were being touched. Well, the bladder has special stretching nerves inside, and when it fills up with urine, these nerves send a signal to your brain telling you it's time to pee. In most cases, the bladder sends its first signal to the brain when it's half full. As it fills up with more and more urine, the signal gets stronger and stronger, telling your brain you really need to pee.

How Does Urine Get Out of the Body?

As you can see in Figures 2-1 and 2-2, urine comes out of your bladder through a tube called the *urethra* (you-REE-thra). In boys, the urethra goes through the penis. In girls, the urethra goes to a small opening right above the vagina. In case you haven't noticed, you don't have to push to get urine out of your body; all you have to do is relax, and your bladder takes care of the rest.

COACH'S CORNER

Why don't children stop playing or watching TV when they need to go to the bathroom?

Parents ask me this question all the time. Although my answer is just a guess, I think lots of kids don't want to be bothered with the basic needs of their bodies. Toddlers don't want to stop playing to get their diapers changed or eat meals. Young children don't want to stop what they're doing to pee or poop. Older kids don't want to come in at night to take a bath. All of this reminds me of a quote by comedian Jerry Seinfeld: "The human body is like a condominium. The thing that keeps you from really enjoying it is the maintenance."

When I was teaching my daughter how to squeeze her sphincter muscle, it reminded me of the Kegel exercises I did after childbirth. Are they related?

When a woman does a Kegel exercise, she's contracting a group of muscles called the pelvic floor. The urethra passes through the pelvic floor, and the sphincter muscle encircles the urethra. The muscles in the pelvic floor do not contract independently from each other. As a result, when you squeeze the sphincter muscle, you contract the entire pelvic floor, including the muscles around the anus. Therefore, from a feeling perspective, contracting one's sphincter muscle is the same as doing a Kegel. (When I describe Kegel exercises to children, I call them pelvic push-ups.)

CHAPTER 3

Why Kids Wet the Bed

When I see children for bedwetting visits, one of the questions I ask is why they think they're wet at night. Here are some of the answers I get.

- "Because I'm a deep sleeper."
- "Because I drink too much after dinner."
- "Because I have a small bladder."

Children usually feel bad about wetting the bed, so I let them know right away that bedwetting is not their fault. Once I'm sure a medical problem isn't causing the wetting (it usually isn't), I tell my patients there's nothing wrong with them either. In most cases, bedwetting occurs because your brain and your bladder aren't "talking to each other" while you sleep. To understand what this means, I need to explain how we learn to be dry at night and what can keep us from reaching this goal.

Learning to Control Your Bladder

Most children become potty trained between 2 and 4 years of age. Children learn to use the potty for a couple of reasons. First, the bladder gets bigger, so it can hold more urine before it fills up. Second, older children develop the ability to hold back urine until they can get to the bathroom. Most kids continue to wear diapers at night even though they use the potty during the

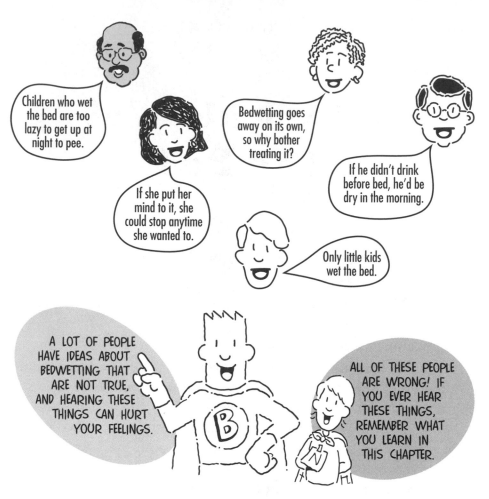

day. The reason kids need diapers at night is because it takes more time for the brain to figure out what the bladder is doing when you're sleeping than when you're awake.

Children usually learn to be dry at night between 3 and 5 years of age. Although some kids get up in the middle of the night to pee, most sleep until morning and go to the bathroom after they wake up. Children learn to be dry at night in 2 steps. First, if the bladder sends a signal to the brain saying that it's filling up with urine, the brain sends a signal back telling the bladder to relax. When the bladder relaxes, it's able to hold more urine, and the child sleeps until morning. Second, if the bladder can't hold all of the urine until morning, it wakes the brain up so you can go to the bathroom and pee. Bedwetting occurs because of a delay in learning these 2 skills.

The final step that leads to a wet bed occurs if your brain doesn't "hear" your bladder in the middle of the night. At first, your bladder says (in bladder talk), "Timmy, I've got to go. It's time to wake up." Your brain doesn't hear the signal.

A little while later, as your bladder fills up with more urine, it says more loudly, "Timmy, I've got to go! It's time to wake up!" Your brain still doesn't hear the signal.

Finally, as your bladder fills up with even more urine, it screams, "TIMMY, I'VE GOT TO GO! IT'S TIME TO WAKE UP!!!" If your brain misses the signal this time, your bladder can't hold the urine anymore and you wet the bed.

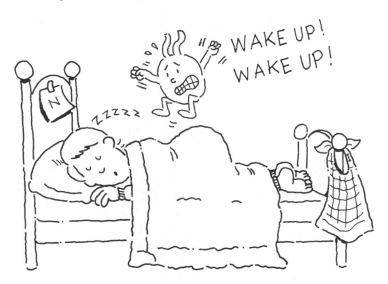

Things That Contribute to Bedwetting

Now that you know how your bladder works, let's discuss some additional facts about bedwetting. Here are the main factors that have an effect on wetting the bed.

Family History

Bedwetting runs in families. Most children who wet the bed have at least one parent (or another close relative) who had the same problem as a child.

Small Bladder

Having a small bladder is one of the main causes of bedwetting. Small bladders don't hold as much urine as normal-sized bladders. Children with small bladders need to pee more often than their friends and sometimes have to run to the bathroom to avoid wetting themselves. When you're sleeping at night, a small bladder is less able to relax and hold all of your urine until morning.

Deep Sleep

Do you remember the experiment on page 16 that explained how the nerves in your bladder send a signal to your brain telling you it's time to pee? Do you remember how you closed your

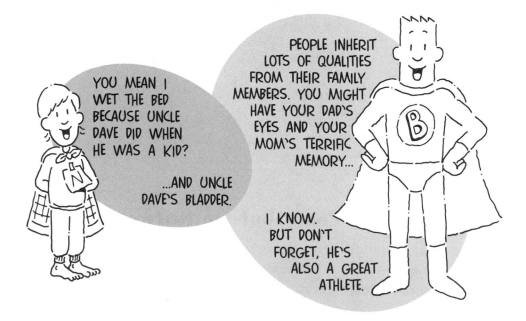

YOU MEAN I WET THE BED BECAUSE UNCLE DAVE DID WHEN HE WAS A KID?

...AND UNCLE DAVE'S BLADDER.

PEOPLE INHERIT LOTS OF QUALITIES FROM THEIR FAMILY MEMBERS. YOU MIGHT HAVE YOUR DAD'S EYES AND YOUR MOM'S TERRIFIC MEMORY...

I KNOW. BUT DON'T FORGET, HE'S ALSO A GREAT ATHLETE.

eyes before your coach touched your hand? You knew instantly
if it was your left or right hand that was being touched. What
do you think would happen if your coach touched your hand
while you were sleeping? Do you think you would wake up or
continue to sleep? Most children would continue to sleep because their brain wouldn't pay attention to a gentle touch while
they were sleeping. However, if someone pinched your hand
while you were asleep, there's a better chance the signal would
get through and you'd wake up. This is similar to what should
happen if your bladder can't hold any more urine at night.
Unfortunately, many children sleep so soundly that they don't
respond to these signals.

Making Too Much Urine at Night

One of the most amazing things about our urinary system is
that the brain and kidney seem to know whether it's day or
night. Because people sleep at night, it would be silly if our kidneys continued to make the same amount of urine as they do
during the day. We'd either need a huge bladder to store it all,
or we'd have to get up 3 times a night to pee. Our bodies figured
out a cool solution to this problem: the brain makes a chemical
at night that tells the kidney to make less urine while we sleep.
Some children don't produce enough of this chemical and wet
the bed because the extra urine overloads their bladders.

Constipation

Constipation is the word we use to describe what happens if
people have poops that are big or hard to pass. If you look at
Figure 2-1 on page 11, you'll see that the *rectum* (RECK-tum)
is right behind the bladder. (The rectum is the place where poop
sits before you go to the bathroom.) If you have a lot of poop in
your rectum, it can push against your bladder and may confuse

the nerve signals that go from your bladder to your brain. This can lead to both daytime wetting and bedwetting. A child may have wetting problems if he has hard poops, large poops or only poops 2 or 3 times a week. *If you're constipated or have infrequent poops, this needs to be corrected before you start the program.* (See the Coach's Corner box on page 26.)

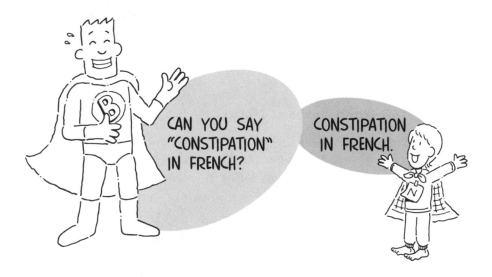

Minor Illness and Fatigue

Being tired or sick doesn't cause bedwetting, but it can trigger episodes of wetting by affecting how you sleep at night. In other words, if you don't feel well, you are less likely to respond to a full bladder when you're sleeping. Although you can't control when you get sick, it's important to go to bed at a reasonable hour so you get a good night's sleep. It also helps if on Friday and Saturday nights you go to bed no more than an hour past your regular bedtime.

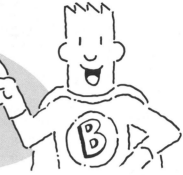

THE AVERAGE 5- TO 9-YEAR-OLD NEEDS 10 TO 11 HOURS OF SLEEP AT NIGHT, AND THE AVERAGE 10- TO 14-YEAR-OLD NEEDS 9 TO 10 HOURS. BY THE TIME KIDS TURN 18, THEY NEED ABOUT 8 HOURS OF SLEEP.

FUN FACT

Depending on where you live, there are many different ways to say, "I have to go to the bathroom." My favorite expression is "I have to go to the can." I thought it would be fun to find out how people refer to bathrooms in different settings and other countries. To test your smarts, match the expression in the left-hand column with the place of origin on the right.

1. The washroom
2. The loo
3. The necessary
4. The head
5. Les toilettes
6. Los servicios
7. Johnny on the spot
8. The dunny
9. Die Toilette
10. Il gabinetto

a. Mexico
b. The Navy
c. Australia
d. Canada
e. Germany
f. Italy
g. England
h. Colonial America
i. France
j. Portable toilet

Correct answers: 1 (d), 2 (g), 3 (h), 4 (b), 5 (i), 6 (a), 7 (j), 8 (c), 9 (e), 10 (f)

COACH'S CORNER

My son is dry when he sleeps at his grandmother's house, but he's almost always wet at home.

It's not uncommon for children to be dry if they sleep at a relative's house. Although this sometimes convinces parents that bedwetting is deliberate, it isn't. When children are dry in this situation, it's because their sleep is somehow altered when they're not in the comfort of their own homes. If you look at this from another perspective, having success away from home is actually reassuring because it shows that your son can be dry at night.

What do you mean when you say that children wet the bed because they have a small bladder?

When children with small bladders are examined under anesthesia, their bladders are actually normal in size. This means the bladder is not anatomically small, but the child has the sensation that the bladder is full before it really is. The medical term for this condition is a *small functional bladder capacity.* I chose the simpler term for kids because it's easier to understand.

My son has a bowel movement every 3 days. I don't understand how this affects his being dry at night.

Infrequent stools (or constipation) can affect bedwetting in a couple of ways. First, as mentioned in the Constipation section on page 23, a full rectum can confuse the nerve signals that are sent to the brain. Second, a full rectum may reduce how much urine the bladder can hold or how well the bladder empties when a child pees. If a child has a bedwetting problem, his bladder will function better if he has a soft or well-formed stool every day.

There are 2 ways to help children have regular stools—diet and medication. The first thing to do is to adjust the diet according to Table 3-1. In many cases, you can achieve success by cutting back on constipating foods rather than asking children to eat foods they don't like. If this doesn't work, talk to your doctor about adding a stool softener to your child's diet. If your child has a more serious problem, such as stool withholding or soiling, you should not do the program without medical supervision (see Appendix B).

Table 3-1.
Foods That Affect Stools

Foods That Make Stools Harder	Foods That Make Stools Softer
• Milk, cheese, and yogurt	• Fruits and vegetables
• White rice, bread, and pasta	• Whole grain rice, bread, and pasta
• Apples and bananas	• Water and juice (Apple is OK.)

One of my friends told me her daughter's bedwetting resolved when she took milk out of her diet.

Although some doctors recommend elimination diets for children who wet at night, there is little research to support this approach. Because many children are picky eaters to begin with, I have not made diet therapy a regular part of my program. There are some foods and beverages that can make a child produce more urine, however, so it's a good idea to avoid these things at dinner. These include chocolate, salty foods, and drinks that contain caffeine (eg, cola, some brands of root beer, tea, coffee).

My 9-year-old snores at night, and one of my friends told me this could cause bedwetting.

There are different ways that children snore. Most of the time, they're just noisy at night, but their breathing is steady and comfortable. Some children have a problem called *obstructive sleep apnea*. Children with this condition not only snore but have difficulty breathing and make intermittent gasping sounds as they try to get air into their lungs. The problem is usually

continued on next page

caused by large adenoids or tonsils. The connection between sleep apnea and bedwetting is unclear, but bedwetting often resolves after children have had surgery to correct their breathing. What's most important here is the apnea, not the bedwetting. If your child has significant snoring at night, you should discuss this with your doctor.

Why does my daughter wet some nights and not others?

I know it seems odd that children can be wet 3 nights in a row, dry for 5 nights, and wet again the following night. No one knows why this happens, but it probably has to do with fluctuations in those factors that make them wet in the first place—how much urine they produce during the night, the ability of their bladders to hold urine, and how easily they arouse from sleep.

My 8-year-old son has attention-deficit/hyperactivity disorder (ADHD). One of my friends told me this would make it harder for him to become dry at night.

Although ADHD does not cause bedwetting, children with attention issues are more likely to wet the bed than other kids. The reason for this association is not clear, but it probably has something to do with the subtle neurologic differences that underlie both conditions. Some authors report that 40% of children with ADHD wet the bed, though this number seems inflated based on my experience.

Over the years, I have successfully treated bedwetting problems in many children with ADHD. Although it's a little more difficult to help these kids, the problems you run into are just what you'd expect—lack of focus, inattention, and impulse control that make it harder for them to stay on task. In addition, some children with ADHD also have learning problems, which can make it harder for them to understand the nuances of the program. Therefore, when I see children with ADHD (or learning disabilities), I make the program as straightforward as possible (see the Coach's Corner box on page 142).

If your child takes medicine for his ADHD, consider giving him a small dose of a quick-acting preparation around 4:00 pm to help him stay focused on the bedwetting program. However, don't change your child's medication without first consulting your doctor.

My husband stopped in our 9-year-old's room the other night before he went to sleep at 11:00 pm. As he peeked in the door, Billy said, "Hi, Dad." Then he urinated in his bed. My husband is convinced our son is too lazy to get out of bed at night.

Billy probably has what we refer to as an arousal disorder. What this means is Billy is unaware of the physical signals his body produces at night. Children like Billy are often described as deep sleepers, but what's really going on is they can't rouse from one sleep state to another.

When Billy said hello to his dad, he was not really awake and had no idea he peed in the bed. Some children think they're in the bathroom when they wet at night. It seems their bladder has roused them just enough to have a vague sense that they need to urinate, but they're not awake enough to know where they are, so they "dream" they're in the bathroom. It's not until they wet the bed that some of them wake up and realize what happened. Other kids don't even wake up when they urinate, or they wake up later in the night (long after the wetting episode) when they're in a lighter state of sleep. The most important thing in this circumstance is that no one makes Billy feel bad for his wetting. The bedwetting alarm and waking up practice are the aspects of the program that address this issue. That's where you should put your energy.

continued on next page

Do psychological problems cause bedwetting?

Although children may develop secondary bedwetting after an episode of emotional stress, psychological problems do not cause primary bedwetting (see Chapter 4 for definitions). Examples of stressful situations that can trigger nighttime wetting include moving to a new home, changing schools, or the death of a loved one. The wetting usually resolves when the stress passes. Keep in mind, however, that bedwetting itself is very stressful for some children and, as a result, can be the cause of anger, social withdrawal, or poor self-esteem.

My sister-in-law says that punishing a child is the best way to stop bedwetting.

Punishing a child for wetting the bed is not something that health care professionals would ever suggest, even though caregivers may resort to this approach out of frustration and anger. Punishment comes in many forms: a child could be grounded for wetting the bed; she could be sent to her room without dessert; or she might be spanked. *Punishment does not cure bedwetting and spanking is never acceptable.* If you have punished your child in the past, tell her you were wrong, and explain to her why you thought it would help. After you have this discussion, a simple apology is in order, not only to make your child feel better but because it cleans the slate before you begin the program.

We're all human, so it's not unreasonable to get frustrated or angry when children are wetting at night or not cooperating with the program. If you find yourself ready to blow, take a deep breath, walk away, and think of another way to vent your emotions. Talk to your spouse, a friend, or a medical professional. If you spend a little time taking care of yourself, you will have more energy to help your child attain her dream of becoming dry at night.

My 8-year-old started wetting the bed 3 weeks after she began taking Zoloft.

Medication occasionally triggers secondary bedwetting. Drugs that have been known to cause this problem include antidepressants such as sertraline hydrochloride (Zoloft), antihistamines, and others. In some cases, changing the time you give the medication or adjusting the dose may control the wetting. Never make an adjustment in any prescription medication without first consulting your doctor, however.

Is there a medication for children who make too much urine at night?

The chemical that reduces urine production at night is called vasopressin. There is a synthetic form of this chemical that helps some children control their bedwetting. I discuss this in more detail in Chapter 27.

Do urinary tract infections cause bedwetting?

Most children who wet the bed have done so for years, and bladder infections are rarely the cause of the problem. If your child suddenly starts bedwetting, a bladder infection may be the cause. Bladder infections are easily discovered when the doctor tests your child's urine.

CHAPTER 4

What Type of Wetting Do You Have?

Now that we've reviewed how your body works and why kids wet at night, let's figure out what type of bedwetting you have. The best way to do this is to ask you some questions about your bladder habits. Before we get to the questions, however, I want to teach you some of the words we use to describe different types of wetting.

- **Nighttime wetting** describes children who wet the bed when they're sleeping. Although most children do this at night, it also applies to children who wet the bed when they're napping.
- **Daytime wetting** describes children who wet themselves when they're awake.
- **Primary wetting** describes children who never learned to be dry at night. They may have had brief periods of dryness, but they were never dry for more than 6 months in a row.
- **Secondary wetting** describes children who were dry for 6 months or more but began wetting again.

Mini-Questionnaire

Before you answer the following questions, I should mention that you can combine bedwetting words in lots of ways. For example, you can have nighttime wetting, daytime wetting, or both. You can have primary nighttime wetting or secondary daytime wetting and so forth. Although this may seem confusing, the type of wetting you have affects how doctors treat you. (Ask your coaches for help if it's too hard to answer Question 4.)

1. Do you wet the bed when you're sleeping? ☐ Yes ☐ No

2. Have you ever been dry at night for
   6 months in a row or more? ☐ Yes ☐ No

3. Do you wet your underpants during the day? ☐ Yes ☐ No
   (If you have damp underpants once or twice a week because you wait too long to go to the bathroom, you should answer no. If your underpants are damp more often or they are actually wet during the day, you should answer yes.)

4. The type of wetting I have is _____.

   Most of the children I see for bedwetting visits have *primary nighttime wetting*. If you have daytime wetting or you started wetting after being dry for 6 months, you should not use the book without your doctor's help.

KID'S ALERT Before you start the program, your coaches need to pay attention to what you do in the bathroom for a couple of days. Please cooperate with them even if it grosses you out a little. The information they collect is very important for the program.

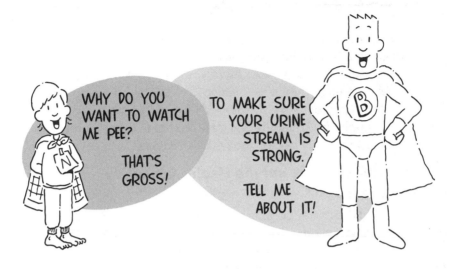

WHY DO YOU WANT TO WATCH ME PEE?

THAT'S GROSS!

TO MAKE SURE YOUR URINE STREAM IS STRONG.

TELL ME ABOUT IT!

COACH'S CORNER

Why do I need to fill out a questionnaire about my son's bowel and bladder habits?

At the end of the introduction, I mentioned that the book is not intended for children with complicated forms of bedwetting. I would like to explain in more detail what I had meant by this statement. Complicated forms of bedwetting have another component that makes them more difficult to treat. Here are some examples.

- A child with daytime and nighttime wetting
- A child with stool soiling and nighttime wetting
- A child with a medical or psychological problem that's causing or directly affecting bedwetting (eg, diabetes, sickle cell disease, certain developmental or psychiatric disorders)

In each of these cases, bedwetting is either secondary to or complicated by another problem, and that problem needs to be addressed before the bedwetting can be treated. Although

continued on next page

the program can still work in these situations, you should get professional help before proceeding. In other words, if you plan to use the book on your own, your child's diagnosis should be primary nighttime wetting. Fortunately, this applies to 85% of children who wet the bed. The Health Screening Questionnaire in Appendix B is designed to uncover medical conditions that your doctor should be aware of.

Is it difficult to fill out the Health Screening Questionnaire?

When kids are little, parents have a pretty good sense of their elimination patterns. Once children reach 5 or 6, most parents fall out of the "poop loop" and are less knowledge-able about what goes on in the bathroom. Before you answer the questions, you should spend a few days observing your child's bowel and bladder habits. Read the questionnaire before you start, and keep a record of your observations so you can answer the questions accurately. A good time to do this is when your child is determining the size of his bladder (see Chapter 8). Be aware that you can't take your child's word for what's happening in the bathroom because kids will often tell you what they think you want to hear. For example, constipated children sometimes "go" every day, but they pro-duce small, hard stools instead of larger ones that are soft or normally formed.

Is there another word doctors use for bedwetting?

Nocturnal enuresis (en-you-REE-sis) is the medical word for bedwetting, and *diurnal* (die-UR-nal) *enuresis* is the medical word for daytime wetting. I use the word *wetting* in the chap-ter because it's easier for kids to understand.

My son only wets the bed once or twice a week. Is he a good candidate for your program?

Someone who wets the bed once or twice a week is proba-bly a year away from becoming dry on his own. In addition, the bedwetting alarm is less successful with these children because they don't wet often enough to learn what the alarm is designed to teach. If your child is motivated to become dry and does all 4 steps of his dry-bed homework (see Chapter 6), there are a few options to consider. First, you can give him a glass of water right before he goes to sleep. This makes it more likely that he will wet the bed and, paradoxically, improves the effectiveness of the alarm. (See overlearning in the Dealing With Relapses section on page 189.) Second, you can do the Modified Waking Up Dry Program on page 79 with or without medication.

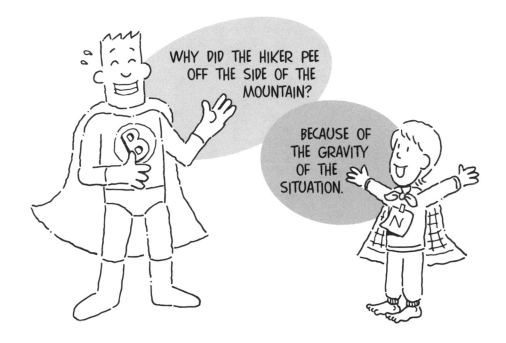

CHAPTER 5

Pop Quiz

OK, kids. It's time to take a break from all the hard work you've been doing. The following quiz reviews some of the basic facts about your body and how you become dry at night. I'm not keeping score, though, so it's not like the tests you take at school. (Circle the correct answers.)

1. Why does your body make urine?
   a. Because it gives you a reason to leave your classroom during the day
   b. So toilets would be invented
   c. Because you need a way to get waste products out of your body

2. What organ in your body makes urine?
   a. Your brain
   b. Your liver
   c. Your kidneys

3. Where are your kidneys located?
   a. In your chest
   b. In your bottom
   c. Behind your intestines

4. Where is urine stored before you go to the bathroom?
   a. In your stomach
   b. In your feet
   c. In your bladder

5. What is your bladder made of?
   a. Skin
   b. Silly Putty
   c. Muscle

6. How many children wet the bed in the United States?
   a. 10,000
   b. 50,000
   c. 5 million

7. Why do children wet the bed?
   a. Because they don't eat their vegetables
   b. Because they watch too much TV
   c. Because they are deep sleepers, have small bladders, or both

8. How do you know when it's time to pee during the day?
   a. Your mom reminds you
   b. You can't stand up anymore because you're trying so hard not to pee in your pants
   c. You feel a tickle or pressure sensation in your bladder

9. Which of the following can contribute to bedwetting?
   a. Eating too much junk food
   b. Forgetting to walk the dog
   c. Constipation

10. Who does most of the work in the Waking Up Dry Program?
   a. Your doctor
   b. Your coach
   c. You

11. Why do some kids run to the bathroom at the last minute when they have to pee?
   a. Because they're having so much fun doing their homework
   b. To drive their parents crazy
   c. Because they ignore their bladder signals until the last second

12. Which of the following is not a reflex action?
   a. Babies peeing in their diaper
   b. Yelling at younger brother and sisters if they pester you
   c. Older kids peeing in the bathroom

13. What's the name of the muscle you squeeze to hold in your urine?
   a. Your biceps
   b. Your gluteus maximus
   c. Your sphincter muscle

14. Does bedwetting run in families?
   a. No
   b. Maybe
   c. Yes

15. What part of your body is responsible for sending bladder signals to your brain?
   a. Your bones
   b. Your tonsils
   c. Your nerves

16. Why do doctors check your urine at bedwetting visits?
   a. To figure out how tall you'll be when you grow up
   b. To see if you're drinking enough milk
   c. To make sure your kidneys and bladder are healthy

17. How is the bladder like a balloon?
   a. They both come in lots of cool colors
   b. They both pop if you fill them up and toss them out
      a window
   c. They both stretch when they fill up with liquid

18. What is the most successful treatment for bedwetting?
   a. Eating tree bark
   b. Staying up late at night
   c. The bedwetting alarm

Answer Key: The correct answer for each question is c.

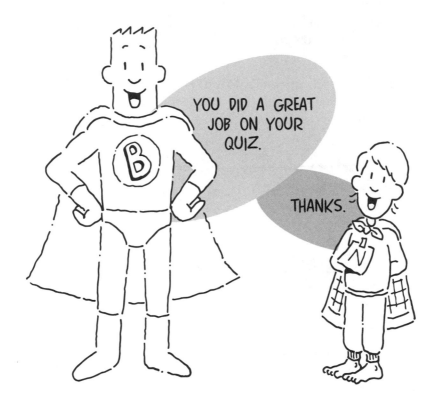

PART 2

Are You Ready to Become Dry?

CHAPTER 6

Dry-Bed Homework

When I see kids for their yearly checkups, I ask them lots of questions. I ask about school. I ask about the foods they eat. I ask if they have any questions about their health. I also ask if they are dry at night. If I find out someone wets the bed, I ask her if she'd like to be dry. This may sound like a silly question, but lots of 4- to 6-year-olds don't mind being wet at night. This is especially true if they wear Pull-Ups to bed. When kids get to be 7 or 8, they almost always want to be dry. There is a big difference, however, between someone who *wants* to be dry and someone who is *ready* to be dry. If a child says she wants to be dry, she may only mean that she wishes her bedwetting would go away. This is similar to wishing you'll get a certain present for your birthday; it's something you want, but you don't have to do anything special to get it. A child isn't ready to be dry until she is willing to do the work it takes to reach that goal. In this chapter, I'm going to help you find out how ready you are to become dry.

Teaching kids about the Waking Up Dry Program requires 2 visits to my office. At the first visit, I find out how often they pee and poop, and I ask about their nighttime wetting. After I talk with them for a while, I do a checkup and have them pee in a cup so I can examine their urine. Once I make sure a medical problem isn't causing their bedwetting, I teach them how their body makes urine and why kids wet the bed at night. At the end of the visit, I give kids a job to do called their dry-bed homework. This homework assignment has 2 goals. First, it gets me

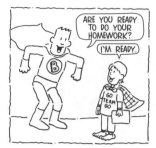 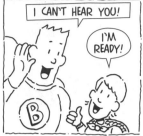 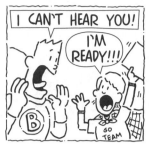

some more information I need for the program. Second, it lets me know how motivated they are to become dry. If a child is interested in the things we discussed and does her homework, I know she's ready to work on the program.

Dry-Bed Homework

Before you start your homework, stop all measures you've been doing to control your bedwetting, including Pull-Ups. That way, you'll get a good picture of your wetting pattern before you start the program. You need to do your homework for *2 weeks* before you score it. The reason for this is that while some steps are performed only once, others need to be done every day. And the best way to test your motivation is to find out if you can stick with something for more than a few days. I'll show you how to score your homework in Chapter 11.

Here is the assignment I want you to do. It's the same one I give to my patients after our first visit.

1. Start paying attention to your bladder. This means you should go to the bathroom as soon as you feel the urge to pee. Also, you should cooperate with your coaches if they ask you to pee before bed or before you leave the house, even if you don't feel the need to go.

2. Make a Waking Up Dry calendar, and record whether you are wet or dry when you get up in the morning (see Chapter 7).

3. Find out the size of your bladder (see Chapter 8).

4. Do the Alarm Clock Test (see Chapter 9).

KID'S ALERT

Continue to read the book while you're doing the dry-bed homework. That way, you'll be ready to start the program as soon as you score your homework.

Sometimes kids prefer to do a few simple things to control their bedwetting instead of doing the regular program. In this situation, we set up an easy version like the one described in Katie's Story below.

Katie's Story

Katie is a 6-year-old who saw me for a checkup a few years ago. During the visit, I found out that Katie wet the bed every night. I knew Katie's wetting was not caused by a medical problem because she was a healthy girl who had no problems with peeing or pooping in the daytime. Katie did not want to wear Pull-Ups anymore, but she got upset if she woke up in a wet bed.

When I described the Waking Up Dry Program, Katie said she preferred doing some easy things to control her bedwetting. This meant she skipped the dry-bed homework and bedwetting alarm. I agreed with Katie's decision, and this is the program we set up. (You can set up the same program as Katie's or work on something different with your coaches.)

continued on next page

Katie's Story, continued

- Katie made a calendar to keep track of her dry nights. Katie decided to call it her *dry-bed calendar.* She also decided she would put stickers on the calendar whenever she had a dry night.
- Katie's mom encouraged her to drink an extra glass of water during the day. Katie liked this idea because her mom said she could have crackers or pretzels with the water.
- Katie agreed to go to the bathroom whenever she felt the urge to pee.
- Every night before she went to sleep, Katie got in bed and her mom reminded her about the tickle feeling that told her it was time to pee. As she lay in bed, she imagined her bladder was filling up like a balloon fills up with water. When she imagined her bladder was as big as an orange, Katie got up and went to the bathroom to pee. As her mom snuggled her in bed, they said the following message together: "If I need to pee at night, I will wake up all by myself and go to the bathroom."
- Katie's mom put underpads (see the Making It Easier to Deal With Wet Bedding section on page 196) on the bed to make cleanup easier in the morning.
- Some days, Katie didn't feel like doing the program. When this happened, her mom did not push the issue.
- Katie's parents gave her a few small rewards for cooperating with the program—an extra book before bed, some extra TV time on the weekend, or a special outing with her mom or dad.

Katie did not become dry right away, but she liked being in charge of her body. After doing her program for a few months, she was dry 3 to 4 nights a week. Katie was very proud of her accomplishment.

COACH'S CORNER

Is it necessary to do the dry-bed homework?

The mainstay of my program is the bedwetting alarm (see Chapter 16), and my goal is to encourage all children 7 years and older to use this device. (I occasionally see 6-year-olds who are motivated enough the use the alarm.) I have learned through experience, however, that many children are not ready to be woken up night after night. I developed the dry-bed homework because it identifies children who are more likely to drop out of the program when the reality of the alarm hits. I think it's better to take a more modest approach with these youngsters than to have them deal with disappointment days or weeks into using the alarm. Articles in medical journals report that up to 25% of children drop out of treatment. My dropout rate is less than 10% because I screen kids before we start.

Can you gauge a child's motivation by the way he approaches his dry-bed homework?

It's important to realize that each child is different. Some children like to talk about becoming dry, and others don't. Some kids ask lots of questions about the program, and others don't. Some kids are hesitant when they try something new, while others dive right in. Some kids are perfectionists and get easily frustrated if things don't work well right away. Some children are more embarrassed about the problem than others, and these kids are usually less interested in talking about their wetting. Also, if parents have punished or reprimanded their child in the past, he may be ambivalent about starting something new. This is equally true for kids who have tried other methods in the past and did not become dry.

You know your child better than anyone, so take that knowledge and apply it to the way he approaches the dry-bed homework. As always, remember to be honest with your child.

continued on next page

When he starts his homework, let him know in an upbeat manner that the way he does these tasks will determine how you proceed with the program. If your child is outwardly enthusiastic and does all of the work, it's easy. If your child is less vocal but still does all of the work, he is probably just as motivated. If you sense some hesitation on your child's part or recognize personality traits that might make things more difficult, be encouraging and see if you can motivate him to do the work. Remind him of past accomplishments and how he succeeded if he stuck with something. You can also say things like, "Jason, it's normal to be unsure of yourself when you're starting something new. But I know you can do it!"

My sister-in-law told me her daughter became dry after one visit to the doctor.

Every few months, I see a child who becomes dry right after our first visit or during the 2 weeks she is doing the dry-bed homework. I'm not sure why this happens, though I suspect the child was close to being dry on her own and paying attention to the problem had nudged her over the fence. Everyone is delighted when this occurs, but I warn parents that the effect may be temporary. If this happens to you, praise your child for her success, but be prepared for a relapse once the **honeymoon period** is over. If she starts wetting again, stay relaxed and pick up where you left off. Let her read this paragraph so she knows it happens to other kids and that it's nothing to worry about. On the other hand, if your child stays dry for 2 weeks, a relapse is unlikely.

My 6-year-old wets the bed 3 times a week. He's not interested in working on becoming dry, but he hides his wet underpants in his closet.

Most children are embarrassed about wetting the bed, and the younger ones often resort to hiding their wet clothes as a means to avoid the problem. Have a nonthreatening discussion with your son about what he's doing. Let him know you understand why he's hiding his underwear but that it's unhealthy to leave wet clothes around the house. If possible, share a secret from your own childhood to help him see you understand what he's going through. In addition, consider giving him some rewards for being more responsible with his wet clothes. This doesn't have to be anything elaborate. Set up a progress chart, and give him a sticker every time he puts his underpants in the laundry basket. When he gets 5 stickers on his chart, let him choose a restaurant for dinner or get some extra TV time. Encourage him to make the chart himself, and make sure you purchase the stickers together.

CHAPTER 7

Waking Up Dry Calendar

When children learn to overcome their bedwetting, they do not become dry right away. Like any other skill, they get better with time. Some children become dry in a few weeks; others take a few months. To follow your progress, it's important to keep a record of wet and dry nights.

Keeping a calendar does a couple of things. First, it lets you know when you reach your goal of being dry 14 nights in a row. Second, because it's easy to get discouraged while you're waiting to become dry, the calendar lets you follow the progress you make along the way. For example, let's say you wet the bed every night before you start the program. Then, by the time you're 4 weeks into it, you're wet every other night. You might be disappointed because you've been doing the program for a long time and you're still wetting the bed. By looking at the calendar, however, you'd see that your wetting has decreased from 7 nights a week to just 3. This is terrific progress, but you wouldn't know it if you didn't keep track of it on your calendar.

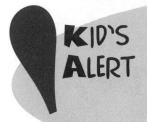

KID'S ALERT The first 2 weeks that you use the calendar is part of your dry-bed homework. Once you begin the program, you will continue to use the calendar to follow your progress.

Setting Up Your Calendar

1. Make or buy a calendar that looks like the one on page 57. This is the best type of calendar to use because you can see a month at a time, which makes it easier to follow your progress. If you decide to buy a calendar, go shopping with your coach so you can pick it out.

    Notice the example on page 57. It shows 3 different ways to mark your calendar. If you have a completely dry night, write *D* for *dry*. If your underpants are wet but the sheets and blanket are dry, write *SW* for *small wet*. If you wet your sheets or blanket in addition to your underpants, write *LW* for *large wet*.

2. I recommend keeping track of large and small wet spots because children usually become dry in stages; they start out with large spots and then have smaller ones until they finally become dry. By keeping a record of both sizes, it's easier to follow your progress. This is especially helpful at the beginning of the program, when it's important to see even small improvements in your wetting.

3. Some kids prefer using stickers or stars when they have dry nights instead of writing *D* on their calendar. If you choose this method, make sure the stickers are small enough to fit inside the space.

4. If you wet more than once a night, you should mark each episode on your calendar.

5. Once you begin the program, it also helps to keep track of your nighttime waking habits. If you wake up on your own when the bedwetting alarm goes off, put a check mark (✓) on your calendar.

6. Keep the calendar in your bedroom because you'll need to fill it in every morning after you wake up. If you forget to mark the calendar, your coaches will remind you to do it.

7. Most children put their calendars in a drawer or closet as soon as they record what happened during the night. If you leave it lying around, you may forget to put it away later. This could be embarrassing if a friend comes over after school and sees the calendar.

8. In the morning, you and your coaches should review whether you were wet or dry during the night.

9. Continue to use your calendar every day you're doing the Waking Up Dry Program.

KID'S ALERT

Some children are very disappointed when they have a wet night. This is especially true if they've been dry for a number of days before they're wet. If this happens to you, you might be tempted to argue with your coaches that the bed was dry. It's important to know that your sheets and underpants may *look* dry in the morning, even though they were wet the night before. Adults are better than kids at seeing urine stains or noticing the smell of urine in your room. Please remember that your coaches want you to be dry as much as you do. If they say you had a wet night, you should believe them.

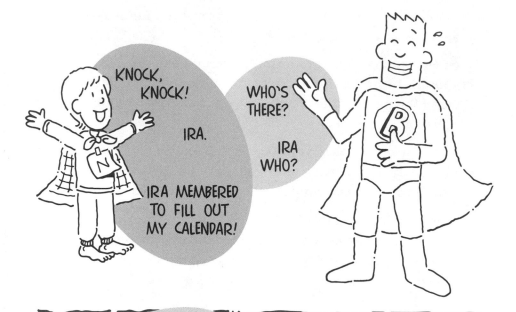

KNOCK, KNOCK!

IRA.

IRA MEMBERED TO FILL OUT MY CALENDAR!

WHO'S THERE?

IRA WHO?

COACH'S CORNER

My 9-year-old daughter appears motivated to work on the program, but she forgets to fill out her calendar.

Children aren't as organized as adults, so this isn't unusual and should not be interpreted as a sign of poor motivation. Ask your daughter if she can think of a way to trigger her memory, such as putting a note on her bathroom mirror or closet door. If she still forgets, remind her to fill out the calendar before she goes to breakfast. Remember that your tone should be encouraging so she doesn't misinterpret your support as nagging.

My son is a little careless at times. What should we do if someone finds his calendar?

This doesn't happen very often, but it's a good idea to have a response handy in case it does (see Chapter 23).

Figure 7-1.
Example of a Completed Waking Up Dry Calendar

July

Sunday	Monday	Tuesday	Wednesday	Thursday	Friday	Saturday
				1 LW	2 LW	3 LW
4 LW ✓	5 LW	6 LW	7 LW ✓	8 SW ✓	9 LW	10 SW ✓
11 SW ✓	12 D	13 SW ✓	14 LW	15 D	16 SW ✓	17 D
18 D	19 SW ✓	20 D	21 D	22 D	23 SW ✓	24 SW ✓
25 D	26 SW ✓	27 D	28 D	29 D	30 D	31 D

✓—Woke up on your own when the bedwetting alarm went off
D—Dry
LW—Large wet
SW—Small wet

57

CHAPTER 8

How Big Is Your Bladder?

By now you know that your bladder is the place where your body stores urine until it's time to pee. I mentioned earlier that some children run to the bathroom at the last minute. Most of the time this happens because kids are too busy watching TV or playing a game to stop what they're doing and go to the bathroom. Some kids have small bladders, however, and they have to pee more often than their friends. The purpose of this chapter is to find out the size of your bladder.

The best way to measure your bladder is to keep a 2-day record of how much you pee each time you go to the bathroom. Although you don't have to stay home the entire time, it helps to do the bladder test on a weekend when you don't have many activities scheduled.

Supplies You'll Need at Home

- A 16-ounce plastic measuring cup
- An index card
- A pen or pencil

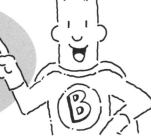

IT HELPS IF YOU DRINK AN EXTRA GLASS OF WATER EACH DAY THAT YOU DO THE BLADDER TEST.

How to Measure Your Bladder

1. Keep a pen or pencil, an index card (see Figure 8-1), and a plastic measuring cup in whichever bathroom you usually use at home.

2. When you feel the urge to pee, go to the bathroom and pee in the cup. Boys usually pee standing up. For girls, it may be easier if you sit on the toilet backwards. This pushes your knees apart and gives you more room to place the cup between your legs. (Your coach can hold the cup if you think it will help.)

3. Record how much urine is in the cup (in ounces) on the index card.

4. Empty the cup into the toilet, and rinse it out.

5. You don't need to record anything if you pee when you're away from home; however, if you're able to hold back your urine, wait until you get home before going to the bathroom.

6. To get an accurate picture of your bladder size, you should pee in the cup more than once. If you don't get 8 to 10 measurements in 2 days, keep the record for an additional day.

Kids sometimes forget to pee in the measuring cup when they're doing the bladder test. You can prevent this from happening by keeping the toilet seat down or by putting a reminder note on the wall behind the toilet. Can you think of some other tricks that will help you remember to pee in the cup?

- _____
- _____
- _____
- _____
- _____
- _____

Figure 8-1.
Example of an Index Card Used to Record Bladder Measurements

Bladder Measurements (in ounces)		
Day 1	**Day 2**	**Day 3 (if needed)**
_____	_____	_____
_____	_____	_____
_____	_____	_____
_____	_____	_____
_____	_____	_____
_____	_____	_____
_____	_____	_____

TIPS & TRICKS

Whenever you go to the bathroom, it's important to empty your bladder completely. Here are some tips to help you accomplish this.

- If you have to go to the bathroom when you're playing a game or watching TV, don't "pee and run." This means you shouldn't rush to get back to what you were doing. Relax and give your bladder a chance to let out all of your urine.
- **For boys.** When you go to the bathroom, pull your underpants all the way down. If you bend your penis over the top of your underpants, it makes it harder for all of your urine to come out.
- **For girls.** When you go to the bathroom, sit back on the toilet seat and separate your legs. If you keep your legs together or sit at the front of the seat, it makes it harder for all of your urine to come out.

How to Tell if Your Bladder Is Small

A child's normal bladder size (in ounces) equals the child's age plus 2. Therefore, the average 6-year-old has a bladder size that is 8 ounces (6 + 2 = 8), while the average 10-year-old has a bladder size that is 12 ounces (10 + 2 = 12). Children who are 12 years and older have a bladder that's the same size as an adult, 12 to 16 ounces. If your bladder measures within 2 ounces of these numbers, it's still considered to be "normal." However, if your bladder is more than 2 ounces below these numbers, you have a small bladder (see Table 8-1).

My largest bladder measurement is _____.

Table 8-1.
Bladder Size According to Age

Age (years)	Normal Range (ounces)	Small Bladder (ounces)
6	6–10	5 or less
7	7–11	6 or less
8	8–12	7 or less
9	9–13	8 or less
10	10–14	9 or less
11	11–15	10 or less
12 and older	12–16	11 or less

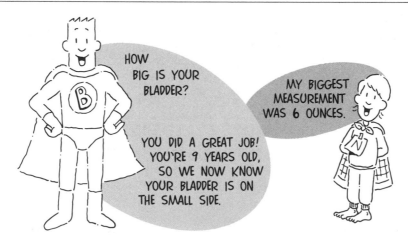

FUN FACT

Have you ever wondered how much urine animals make? Because mammals have bladders, they pee just like people do. Well, not just like people, because they pee on the ground instead of in a toilet. Here's a list of some popular mammals and the amount of urine they make each day.

For comparison purposes, the average human makes about 4 cups (¼ gallon) per day.

- Elephant   208 cups (13 gallons)
- Cow   72 cups (4½ gallons)
- Horse   24 cups (1½ gallons)
- Pig   12 cups (¾ gallon)
- Sheep   8 cups (½ gallon)

If you compare these numbers, you'll find that an elephant produces as much urine in one day as 3 cows, 9 horses, 18 pigs, 26 sheep, or 52 humans. That's a lot of pee!

COACH'S CORNER

Is there any reason to know my son's bladder size, other than finding out if he's willing to cooperate with the program?

In the past, doctors taught children with small bladders to do stretching exercises to try and make their bladders bigger. This treatment isn't recommended anymore because it's hard for children to hold back their urine and current research doesn't support this approach. That said, there are 3 reasons why it's worth knowing if a child has a small bladder.

- It's more important for these children to drink water during the day.
- Children with small bladders are less likely to respond to the medication desmopressin (see Chapter 27).
- Children with small bladders sometimes wet the bed more than once a night. If this happens, they may need to add a medication such as oxybutynin to the program (see the Your Child Wets the Bed More Than Once per Night section on page 183). *continued on next page*

My son has a small bladder, but his teacher doesn't like it if students leave class day after day to use the bathroom.

As every parent knows, there's no shortage of rules at school. Despite all the regulations, you do have one trump card to play—a note from your doctor. I have patients with small bladders who need to visit the bathroom as soon as they feel the urge to go. I have other patients with daytime wetting who need to urinate every 2 hours (they wear a special vibrating wristwatch that discretely reminds them to go). As long as I write a note describing their medical need, schools cooperate with my request.

Your focus seems to be on children with small bladders. My daughter has a large bladder, but she still wets the bed.

Because a large bladder capacity is atypical for children with nighttime wetting, your daughter should be examined for constipation or other problems that interfere with normal bladder emptying.

If her evaluation is normal, there are a few strategies you can incorporate into the program. First, it's important she urinates regularly during the day. She should go to the bathroom every 2 hours even if she doesn't feel the need to pee. The reason for this is because children with large bladders don't appreciate bladder fullness the way most people do. In addition, regular bathroom habits may retrain her bladder over time and allow it to function more normally. I would also suggest she urinates twice before she goes to sleep; have her go 30 minutes before she gets into bed and again right before she turns off the light. Finally, it's important that she follows the advice in the Tips & Tricks box on page 61and remains in the bathroom for a few minutes to give her bladder time to empty.

CHAPTER 9

Alarm Clock Test

The bedwetting alarm is the most effective treatment for learning to be dry at night. However, as I mentioned in the introduction, it also takes the most work. Because lots of kids are deep sleepers, we need to find out if you will wake up when the alarm goes off. The Alarm Clock Test is designed to answer that question.

It takes 3 nights to do the test. On the first night, set the alarm to go off 1 hour after you go to sleep. On the second night, set the alarm to go off 2 hours after you go to sleep. On the third night, set the alarm to go off 3 hours after you go to sleep. You pass the test if you wake up on your own *or* with your coach's help on any of the 3 nights. If you're unable to wake up or you are too sleepy to follow the steps listed in the How to Do the Alarm Clock Test section on the next page, you're not ready to use the bedwetting alarm.

It's common for children not to wake up on their own when they begin using the bedwetting alarm, and the same thing may occur during the Alarm Clock Test. So don't be discouraged if you're too sleepy at first; that's why the test runs for

MAKE SURE YOU HAVE TO GET OUT OF BED TO SHUT OFF THE ALARM; THAT WILL KEEP YOU FROM TURNING IT OFF AND GOING RIGHT BACK TO SLEEP.

3 nights. Also, don't do the test after a really hectic day because it will be harder for you to wake up that night.

Supplies You'll Need at Home

• An electric clock with a buzzing alarm
• A wet washcloth

How to Do the Alarm Clock Test

1. Get ready for bed the way you normally do. Change into your pajamas or nighttime underpants, brush your teeth, and put on your night-light if you use one.

2. If you have never used an alarm clock before, your coach will show you how it works. Your coach can set the alarm, but *you* need to be the one to turn it off after it starts to buzz.

3. Before you go to sleep, practice turning off the alarm. Lie down in bed and pretend to be asleep. Have your coach fast-forward the time so the alarm goes off. Wake up from your pretend sleep and quickly turn off the alarm. Go to the bathroom to pee and return to your room.

4. As you fall asleep, tell yourself that you will pay attention to the alarm and you will wake up as soon as it goes off. Remind yourself that you are the boss of your body!

5. Your coach should go to your room a few minutes before the alarm is set to go off.

6. If you wake up when the alarm goes off, sit up and quickly turn it off. Go to the bathroom to pee. Then go back to sleep.

7. If you don't wake up after the alarm has been buzzing for 10 seconds, your coach will begin the wake-up drill to help you get up.

How to Do the Wake-up Drill

1. Your coach will call your name and say the wake-up message: "Maggie, you need to wake up! Wake up, Maggie! Maggie, you can do it! You need to wake up if you want to have dry beds!" (**Coach's Tip:** Your tone and attitude should be animated and encouraging.)

2. If you don't wake up, your coach will gently shake your shoulders a few times and repeat the wake-up message.

3. If you still don't wake up, your coach will sit you up in bed and repeat the wake-up message.

4. If you still don't wake up, your coach will wet your face with a washcloth and repeat the wake-up message.

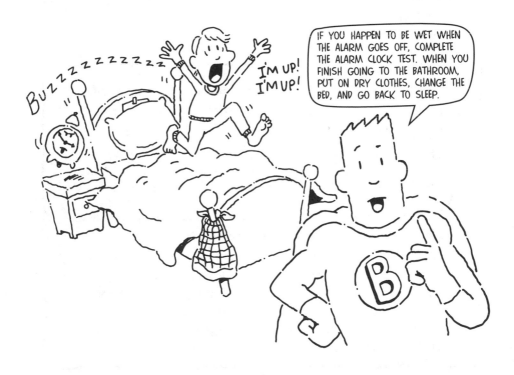

5. If you still don't wake up, your coach will repeat the wake-up message and walk you around the room. (**Coach's Tip:** If you're not strong enough to walk your child around the room, stand her up by the side of the bed. If this is too difficult, skip this step. I don't want anyone to get hurt by falling on the floor.)

6. If you wake up at any point during Steps 1 to 5, you should quickly turn off the alarm. Go to the room to pee. Then go back to sleep.

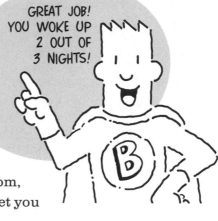

GREAT JOB! YOU WOKE UP 2 OUT OF 3 NIGHTS!

7. If you don't wake up or you are unwilling to turn off the alarm and go to the bathroom, your coach will turn it off and let you go back to sleep.

COACH'S CORNER

How hard should I shake my child when I try to wake him up at night?

Not hard. Think of it as rocking him back and forth with a gentle motion. Some parents find that tickling their children is more effective than shaking them.

Is it important for children to be fully awake when they do the Alarm Clock Test?

Children do not need to be fully conscious when they do the Alarm Clock Test. However, they should be awake enough to turn off the alarm and go to the bathroom. If your child is groggy, you can guide her through each task, if necessary. Stay close by to ensure she gets to and from the bathroom safely.

CHAPTER 10

Family Matters

In Chapter 6, we discussed your readiness to become dry at night. Now we need to look at your family to make sure nothing at home will affect your chances of becoming dry. Here are some things to consider before you begin the program.

Vacation

There are 2 reasons why summer can be a good time to do the program: you can usually sleep later in the morning, and you don't have homework or tests to worry about. Despite these advantages, there is one thing about the summer that can make it harder to work on becoming dry—family vacations. If you're planning to go away in the next 2 months, consider delaying the program until your trip is over.

Moving to a New Home

If you're planning to move in the next month, hold off on starting the program until you're settled in your new home.

Illness

If anyone in the family is scheduled to have an operation or is sick with more than a simple problem, consider delaying the program. Your coaches may be distracted at such times, and they're less likely to be able to give you the attention you need.

Brothers and Sisters

Because most of us have siblings (brothers or sisters), certain
events can make it harder for the program to work. Here are
some things to keep in mind.

- Is your mom about to have a baby?
- Is your family about to adopt a baby?
- Are there 2 children at home who wet the bed? If the answer
  to this question is yes, only 1 person should be treated at a
  time. Logically, the older child should have the chance to
  go first.

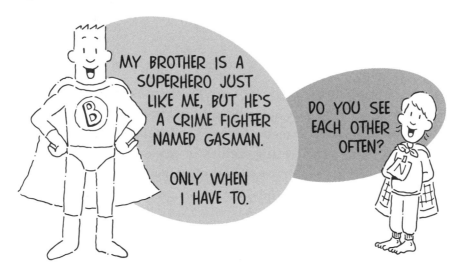

MY BROTHER IS A SUPERHERO JUST LIKE ME, BUT HE'S A CRIME FIGHTER NAMED GASMAN.

ONLY WHEN I HAVE TO.

DO YOU SEE EACH OTHER OFTEN?

Arguing at Home

This is a hard one to discuss, but if you get angry easily or
you and your parents are arguing a lot about homework or
other issues, this may not be a good time to start the program.
Learning to become dry takes a lot of cooperation between you
and your coaches, so if you're already fighting with each other,
the chances are pretty good that you'll fight about the program
too. It's important to note, however, that a little arguing in

families is *normal.* If you have some issues to deal with, this does not mean you can't work on becoming dry. It just means you shouldn't do the program alone with your parents. Work with your doctor or even consider seeing a psychologist (a talking doctor) to help you and your parents work things out.

Family Stress

It's important for the home environment to be supportive and relatively stress free for the program to work. Therefore, if your parents are under a lot of pressure, this may not be a good time to do the program. If only one of your parents is under stress and the other one is available to help you, you can go ahead.

COACH'S CORNER

I have a 4-year-old who wants to stop wearing Pull-Ups. Unfortunately, he's still wet at night, and my husband and I don't know what to do.

Although a 4-year-old is too young to be called a bedwetter, you should respect his wishes to stop wearing Pull-Ups. Children who don't want to use Pull-Ups feel like they're still in diapers, and wearing them can have a negative effect on their self-esteem. In this situation, either protect the bedding to make your laundry chores easier (see Chapter 26) or buy special underwear that can hold large amounts of urine.

My daughter is jealous over the attention her brother is getting with the program.

To start with, tell your daughter you're working on a very important program to help your son overcome his bedwetting.

continued on next page

You can then do 1 of 2 things to enlist your daughter's help. The first choice is to reward her for being supportive. Just as your son gets to pick out weekly rewards for his efforts (see Chapter 14), your daughter can get some token rewards for encouraging her brother. This has to be acceptable with your son, however, because children may not want siblings to say anything about their bedwetting. Alternatively, you can set up a program with your daughter in which she can earn her own rewards. For example, she can get rewards for cleaning up the house (not regular chores, something extra) or working on one of her own problems, such as thumb-sucking.

I have a 9-year-old daughter who wets the bed, and she doesn't want her brother to know about the program.

This is a little tricky, as everyone is living under the same roof. You should respect your daughter's wishes and try to come up with some practical solutions. Here are a few things that may help.

- Don't talk about the problem if her brother is nearby.
- Find a safe place to keep the book and her Waking Up Dry calendar.
- Make sure her brother is doing something when wet bedding is taken to the laundry room (see Alice's Story on page 133).
- If your daughter goes to sleep after her brother, do waking up practice (see Chapter 12) once he's in bed. If she goes to sleep before him, shut her door when she does the exercise and use a chair in her room as a pretend toilet. This will be easier to accomplish if another parent is in charge of her brother.
- If your daughter uses the bedwetting alarm, it will be hard to keep her brother in the dark, even though most siblings don't wake up when the alarm goes off. Just be as discreet as possible, following the same timing advice suggested for waking up practice.

I have an 8-year-old who wets the bed, and I recently found out his 10-year-old brother has been threatening to tell his friends about it.

This is a serious situation. Both parents need to sit down with your older son to work this out. Try to avoid any anger or accusations at the beginning of your talk. Let your son know you found out what's been happening, and ask him to explain his side to you. The bottom line, however, is that this behavior is unacceptable, and you need to convey this to your son. Be very specific about this, and let him know exactly what the consequences will be if he continues to threaten his brother. One final thought: if there are long-standing relationship issues between your children, you should consider seeing a mental health professional to work on the problem.

I was getting ready to start a bedwetting program with my 10-year-old, but his younger brother is having a lot of trouble at school.

There's no such thing as a stress-free home, and the word *multitasking* must have been invented for parents. The question you should ask yourself is whether or not you can devote energy to both of your children at this time. The bedwetting program usually takes 2 to 3 months to complete, with a fair dose of sleepiness thrown in. If you think you can work through your other son's problem more quickly, put the bedwetting program on hold for a while.

My 11-year-old daughter wants to use the bedwetting alarm, but our family situation isn't right for the alarm at the moment. What would you recommend?

If your daughter is motivated to work on her bedwetting, consider an approach she can do independently.

continued on next page

- Have your daughter set her alarm clock to go off an hour before she usually wets the bed. When the alarm goes off, she can get up and go to the bathroom on her own. If she has a history of wetting more than once a night, buy a clock that has 2 alarm settings. Remember, put the clock away from her bed so she has to get up to turn it off.
- If your daughter has trouble waking up at night, she may have more success with a clock that's designed for heavy sleepers. The Wake Assure alarm clock buzzes, flashes a bedside lamp, and vibrates the bed in an effort to accomplish this task. You can buy this clock online.
- Have your daughter do the Modified Waking Up Dry Program described on page 79.
- Ask your doctor about using the medication desmopressin (see Chapter 27). If this is ineffective or only provides short-term relief, you can reconsider the bedwetting alarm at some point in the future.

My husband and I are divorced. Does this mean my son can't do the program?

If parents are divorced or separated, the program is obviously more difficult to do. Here are some questions to ask yourself before you begin.

- Can you communicate with your ex-husband?
- Does your son see his father regularly?
- Do you and your ex-husband agree on doing the program?
  If you and your ex-husband can communicate with each other, it's OK to proceed. It's important that both of you to follow the program the same way, however. If you disagree about certain aspects of the program, discuss this with your child's doctor. Also, make sure your son has his calendar and other materials when he travels from one home to the other.

PART 3

Getting Set for the Program

CHAPTER 11

Scoring Your Dry-Bed Homework

When I work with children in my office, I meet with them 2 weeks after our first visit. At this time, I review their dry-bed homework and we set up the program. Because I won't be meeting with you 2 weeks after you do your homework, you'll need another way to do this. If you're doing the program with your doctor, he or she can help you build the program. If you're doing the program at home, your coaches will help.

It's important to be honest when you score your home-work and to remember that your coaches need to agree with you about how things went. For example, the hardest part is the Alarm Clock Test. Sometimes children are very sleepy when the alarm goes off, and they won't get up, even when their coaches do the wake-up drill. Then, the following morning, they don't remember what happened and think everything

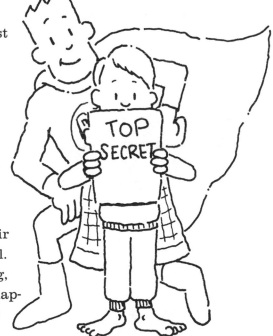

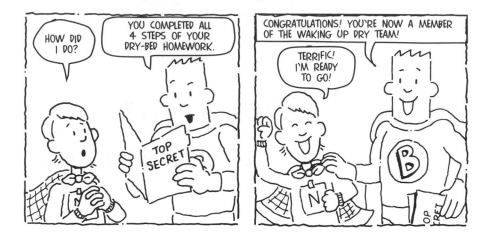

went well. Keep in mind that your coaches want you to be dry as much as you do, and adults remember what happens at night better than kids. So if your coaches tell you Step 4 didn't go well, you should believe them.

Scoring Your Homework

If you weren't able to complete the first 3 steps of the dry-bed homework, you're not ready to do the program. There are still a few things you can do to help yourself, however, so consider the following options:

- Read Katie's Story on page 47. If you like her program, you can do all or part of this yourself.
- If you're younger than 8 years and don't want to do anything about your wetting, it's OK if you use Pull-Ups at night. Older children should not use Pull-Ups except in special circumstances (see Chapter 24).
- Talk to your coaches about having one of them take you to the bathroom right before they go to sleep. This is called *lifting* and is discussed in Chapter 24.

If you completed the first 3 steps of the dry-bed homework but not the fourth, you're not ready to use the bedwetting alarm, but like Katie (see page 47), you can do a number of things to help yourself become dry (I call this the Modified Waking Up Dry Program).

The Modified Waking Up Dry Program

1. Fill out your Waking Up Dry calendar every day, keeping track of wet and dry nights.

2. Do the waking up practice every night as described in Chapter 12.

3. Do the bladder exercises as described in Chapter 13.

4. If you don't make any progress after a few months, you can redo the Alarm Clock Test to see if you're ready to use the bedwetting alarm.

5. If you're still not ready to use the bedwetting alarm, add lifting to the program (see Chapter 24) or talk to your doctor about taking a medication to reduce your nighttime wetting (see Chapter 27).

If you completed all 4 steps of the dry-bed homework, you're ready to do the regular program. The next few chapters describe the bedwetting alarm and some extra things you can do that help kids become dry. I will show you how to set up the program in Chapter 20.

COACH'S CORNER

My son is disappointed because he really wanted to use the bedwetting alarm, but he didn't wake up when we did the Alarm Clock Test.

Although the Alarm Clock Test is a good measure of a child's ability to respond to the bedwetting alarm, you have a few more options at this point. First, tell your son his cooperation earned him another shot at the test. This time, do it for 5 nights instead of 3. If he's still unable to awaken, remind him that lots of kids are deep sleepers and that his ability to wake up will improve as he gets older. In the meantime, be enthusiastic about the modified program described on the previous page.

Second, you can consider using the bedwetting alarm even though he didn't wake up to the alarm clock. I have had a handful of patients over the years who become dry with the bedwetting alarm even though they did not pass the Alarm Clock Test. In some cases, they began waking up a few weeks into using the alarm. In others, they never woke up when the alarm went off but began having fewer wet nights and eventually became dry. If you try this approach, keep in mind that it will be harder to deal with your child's wet bed in the middle of the night.

My 8-year-old has been doing the Modified Waking Up Dry Program for 2 months. She started out wetting the bed every night and now wets 3 or 4 times a week. We tried the Alarm Clock Test, but she was too sleepy to get up. She's still doing the program, but her enthusiasm isn't what it used to be.

Although I can appreciate your daughter's frustration, she's made great progress, considering she used to wet the bed every night. I mentioned previously that the bedwetting alarm is the most successful treatment for bedwetting. The cure rate for the modified program isn't as good. These children become dry or reduce their wetting frequency 40% to 50% of the time. (See the Coach's Corner box on page 115 for statistics on the bedwetting alarm.)

There are a few ways you can handle this situation.

- Continue with the modified program. In time, your daughter may have more dry nights per week. If you take this approach, tell her she's doing very well and to keep up the good work. You should also consider talking to your doctor about adding a medication to the program.

- Stop the program. If you take this approach, tell your daughter she's done a great job so far, but sometimes it helps to take a breather for a while. You can restart the modified program in 6 to 12 months or redo the Alarm Clock Test to see if she's ready for the bedwetting alarm.

CHAPTER 12

Waking Up Practice

Most children become dry at night because their bladders learn to hold all of their urine until morning. Others need to wake up if their bladders get full while they're sleeping. Therefore, one of the things that will help you become dry is to learn to wake up if your bladder signals your brain that it can't hold any more urine. Waking up practice is an exercise that helps accomplish this task.

Before you do waking up practice, get ready for bed the way you normally do. Change into your pajamas or nighttime underpants, and turn on your night-light. If you don't use a night-light, you'll need another source of light so you can see what you're doing in the middle of the night. Here are some other options.

• A lamp with a low-wattage bulb
• A ceiling light with a dimmer switch
• A bathroom or hallway light that provides enough brightness in your room

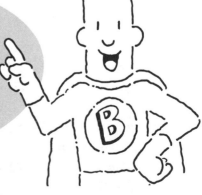

WHEN YOU PEE AT NIGHT, REMEMBER TO STAY IN THE BATHROOM LONG ENOUGH TO EMPTY YOUR BLADDER COMPLETELY.

How to Do Waking Up Practice

1. Lie in bed, close your eyes, and pretend you're asleep.

2. Imagine your bladder is the size of a lemon.

3. Imagine your bladder is filling up with urine. As your bladder fills up, it gets bigger like a balloon filling up with water.

4. Imagine your bladder is now the size of an orange. At this size, it sends a signal to your brain telling you it's time to pee. Concentrate on this feeling.

5. Imagine the tickle or the pressure sensation you get during the day when you need to pee, only now the feeling is stronger, much stronger.

6. Imagine your bladder is telling your brain it's time to wake up. You need to wake up so you can go to the bathroom and pee. You need to wake up so you will be dry in the morning.

7. Imagine you are waking up. Open your eyes and quickly squeeze your sphincter muscle to make sure you stay dry. (See the Hands On box on page 15 for a reminder of how to do this.)

8. Get out of bed, go to the bathroom, and pee.

9. Go back to your room and lie down. Feel your sheets and imagine waking up in a nice dry bed. Remind yourself that you are going to wake up if your bladder can't hold all of your urine until morning.

10. Remind yourself that you are the boss of your bladder.

Your coach should read the 10 steps to you every night for the first week you're doing the program. (This lets you concentrate on the feelings I describe in the exercise.) After the first week, you can do waking up practice on your own if you're an experienced reader. First, read the steps to yourself before you get in bed. Then, turn off your light and use your imagination to follow the steps outlined in the exercise. If you are a younger

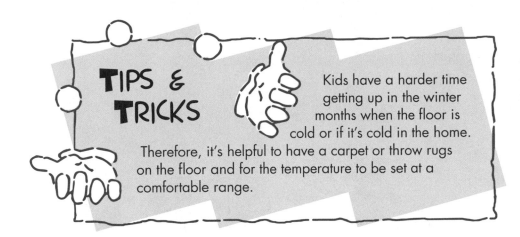

TIPS & TRICKS

Kids have a harder time getting up in the winter months when the floor is cold or if it's cold in the home. Therefore, it's helpful to have a carpet or throw rugs on the floor and for the temperature to be set at a comfortable range.

reader, your coach can continue to read the steps until you remember them.

Even if you're a terrific reader, consider having your coach read the 10 steps to you once a week so you can concentrate on how your bladder feels when it fills up at night. (This is an optional part of the program, so you don't have to do it if you don't want to.)

Darrell's Story

I saw a 7-year-old a few years ago who came up with an interesting idea for his waking up practice. Darrell wanted to do the exercise on his own, even though he was just learning to read. Instead of having his coach read the exercise to him at night, he asked his dad to record the 10 steps on a cassette. (Nowadays, you would use a cell phone or an electronic recorder.) When Darrell got into bed, he played his dad's tape so he could concentrate on how his bladder would feel when it was trying to wake him up at night. He thought about the way his bladder filled up with urine when he slept. He thought about how his bladder would send a signal to his brain trying to wake him up. And he got up and practiced going to the bathroom to pee. The tape worked perfectly, and Darrell was proud of his ability to do things on his own.

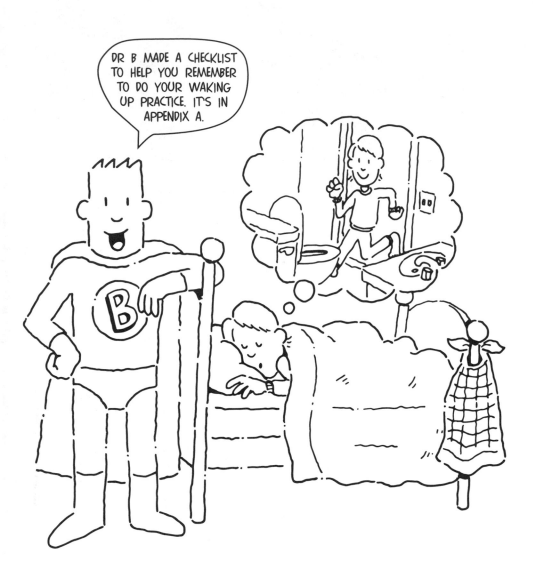

COACH'S CORNER

My daughter is afraid of the dark. Will this interfere with getting up at night to use the bathroom?

Fear of the dark and not wanting to get up when it's cold are the most common reasons children are reluctant to use the bathroom at night. I already discussed how to handle cold nights in the Tips & Tricks box on page 85. The best way to deal with fear of the dark is to use a night-light or leave a child's ceiling light on (a dimmer switch will enable you to lower the light intensity to a reasonable level). If adding light to the room isn't enough, consider the following options:

- Put a portable potty in your daughter's room while she's working on the program.
- Tell your daughter she can call you at night if she needs someone to go with her to the bathroom. Although this is clearly inconvenient for parents, it's worth doing if it gives your daughter the confidence she's looking for to enable her to overcome her bedwetting.

My son has been doing the program for 2 weeks. Last night, he said he didn't need to do his waking up practice anymore.

Your son may be right or, more likely, he is feeling overwhelmed with how much he has to do to become dry at night. Don't get into a power struggle over this issue. Instead, ask him if he thinks the exercise is too much for him to do at this point. If he says yes, let him know his input is important and it's OK to stop this part of the program for a while. You might gently suggest restarting the exercise in the future if you think it would be helpful.

CHAPTER 13

Bladder Exercises

By now you know that the bladder plays a big role in keeping kids dry at night. As a result, one of the things that will help you become dry is to exercise your bladder during the day. This chapter describes 2 exercises. The first one helps your bladder hold more urine. The second one helps you become more aware of your bladder signals when you need to pee.

Water Gulping

Over the years, I've learned that lots of kids don't drink much during the day. For example, many children skip breakfast and eat lunch without drinking more than a few sips of water or juice. One of the things that happens if you don't drink is you make less urine. And if you make less urine, your bladder may

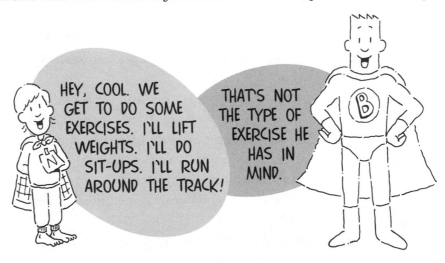

HEY, COOL. WE GET TO DO SOME EXERCISES. I'LL LIFT WEIGHTS. I'LL DO SIT-UPS. I'LL RUN AROUND THE TRACK!

THAT'S NOT THE TYPE OF EXERCISE HE HAS IN MIND.

lose its ability to hold urine at night. Therefore, the best thing you can do to exercise your bladder is drink more during the day. (I call this exercise water gulping.) By drinking more, your bladder fills up more often and you get more practice going to the bathroom to pee. Water gulping also changes the way you drink. Many children drink most of their liquids at dinner or before bed. Water gulping encourages you to drink earlier in the day. (If you normally drink a lot of liquids, you can skip this exercise.)

How to Do Water Gulping

1. Drink 2 extra glasses of water during the day.
2. Drink the first glass with lunch and the second glass when you come home from school. (If you usually have milk or juice with lunch that can count as one of your drinks, as long as you finish it.)
3. If it's a nonschool day, drink the first glass with lunch and the second glass sometime before dinner.
4. Because it's hard to change the way you drink, it will help if you keep a water gulping chart. One way to do this is to use the checklist in Appendix A. In addition, consider the following suggestions:
   • Put a reminder note (or bottle of water) in your lunch box.
   • If you use a homework journal, write a reminder note in it.
   • Leave a bottle of water on the kitchen table or other places you're likely to go when you first get home from school.
   • Have one of your coaches remind you to drink some water when you get home from school. (Your coaches should not do this unless you give them permission to remind you.)
   • Water is more enjoyable if you drink it with a salty snack, such as pretzels or crackers.
5. Continue the exercise as long as you're doing the program.

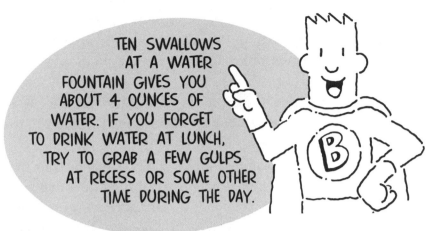

TEN SWALLOWS AT A WATER FOUNTAIN GIVES YOU ABOUT 4 OUNCES OF WATER. IF YOU FORGET TO DRINK WATER AT LUNCH, TRY TO GRAB A FEW GULPS AT RECESS OR SOME OTHER TIME DURING THE DAY.

Bladder Attention

I mentioned in Chapter 3 that the reason kids wet the bed is because their bladders and brains aren't talking to each other at night. One way to help this process is to think about your bladder signals during the day. If you pay close attention to these feelings, it may help your brain recognize them while you're sleeping. (I call this exercise bladder attention.)

How to Do Bladder Attention

1. As soon as you feel the urge to pee, stop what you're doing and go to the bathroom.
2. Think about how your stretching nerves are sending a signal to your brain, letting you know it's time to pee.
3. Remind yourself that these are the same signals your bladder sends to your brain while you're sleeping.
4. Picture your bladder filling up like a balloon fills up with water.
5. When you get to the bathroom, imagine your bladder is the size of an orange and concentrate on this picture as you start to pee.

6. Remember the tips in the Tips & Tricks box on page 61 that make it easier for your bladder to let out all of your urine.

7. After you finish peeing, squeeze your sphincter muscle a couple of times. Remember that this is the muscle you use to hold in your urine.

8. Do this exercise 2 or more times per day. The best time to do it is in the morning before school or in the afternoon when you get home. On nonschool days, do it anytime you're home.

9. It will help you remember to do the exercise if you make a chart and record each time you do it. One way to do this is to use the checklist in Appendix A.

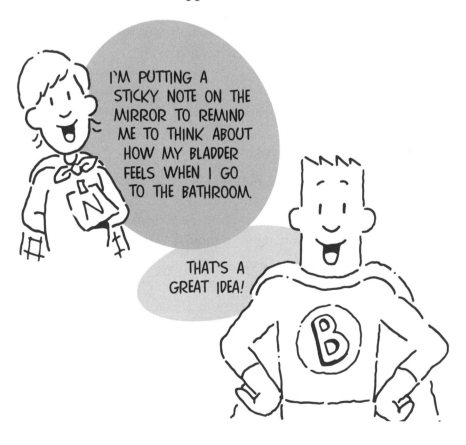

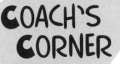

COACH'S CORNER

My 9-year-old drinks three 8-ounce glasses of water or juice every day. Does he need to do water gulping?

I mentioned in the Water Gulping section on page 90 that kids can skip this exercise if they drink a lot during the day. From what you've mentioned, it sounds like your son is drinking plenty of fluids on his own. Therefore, it's not necessary for him to add water gulping to the program. Give him a thumbs-up, and tell him to keep up the good work.

My daughter doesn't want to do water gulping because it makes her urinate more during the day, and she doesn't like using the bathroom at school.

I hear about this almost every day at work, not the water gulping part but the part about children not wanting to use the bathroom at school. When I ask kids why they're reluctant to use the bathroom, here are the answers I get.
- "The toilet seats are wet."
- "There's no privacy."
- "It's too smelly."
- "The room is gross."
- "I just don't want to."

There are 2 ways to address your daughter's concerns. The first is trying to convince her to use the bathroom. The second is adjusting the program to fit her needs. Here is a list of some things she can do to make the bathroom experience more tolerable.
- Show her how adults use toilet paper to dry and cover toilet seats before they sit down.
- Show her how you can squat over a toilet to pee.
- Have her use the bathroom during class time when fewer kids are there. This may require a note for the teacher letting the school know your daughter has a bladder problem.

continued on next page

- Ask if she can use the bathroom in the nurse's office.

If these ideas don't change your daughter's mind, you'll need to adjust the water gulping exercise. The obvious solution is to drink 1 glass of water after school and 2 glasses per day on weekends and holidays.

My son has trouble doing his bladder attention exercise because he has a small bladder and needs to pee as soon as he feels the urge to go.

Children with small bladders often have little warning before they urinate, and when they get the urge to go, it's very strong and difficult to inhibit. (Kids with normal-sized bladders will have the same sensation if they wait until the last minute to go.) Tell your son not to worry if he doesn't have time to think about how his bladder feels. Have him focus on getting to the bathroom as soon as he feels the urge to go. He can then imagine his bladder getting smaller as he urinates.

My daughter forgot to do her water gulping for the past 2 days. I want to remind her, but I don't want to nag.

Because I've been helping kids become dry for many years, I know it's hard to do these exercises every day. Sometimes a child may forget to do them. Other times a day may be too complicated to fit everything in. Remind your daughter that the exercises are important, but it's OK if she misses them once in a while. Then suggest you sit down to discuss the situation. If you work on the problem together, she is more likely to interpret your help in a positive way rather than as nagging.

CHAPTER 14

Contracts & Rewards

The purpose of this chapter is to explain why you sign a contract before you begin the program and why I think it's a good idea to give you rewards for the work you put into becoming dry at night. The contract and types of rewards I'm referring to are described in Chapter 21.

What Is a Contract?

A contract is an agreement between people that puts into writing something they say they will do. It's common for grown-ups to sign contracts before they begin a project. For example, if someone is painting your house or installing a new air conditioner, your parents will sign a contract that says what's going to be done and how much it will cost.

Why Do I Need to Sign a Contract Before Doing the Waking Up Dry Program?

A lot of kids aren't sure why they need to sign a contract before they start using their alarm. We do this because the program may last for a few months, and it's easy to forget what you agreed to do before you started. By putting things into a contract, you and your coaches will know exactly what's expected during the program. This makes it less likely that you will argue about things later on.

What Are Rewards?

My grandfather used to say the best reward is the satisfaction one gets from accomplishing something. For example, let's say you've been practicing a new song on the piano for weeks. You practice for 30 minutes every day. In the beginning, you make lots of mistakes; either you hit the wrong keys, or your timing is off and the song doesn't sound the way you want it to. Whenever you sit down to play, you get frustrated because your fingers won't do what you want them to do. Your parents and piano teacher encourage you and reassure you that you will master the song in time. In the beginning, you can't imagine that you will ever learn the song. However, by practicing day after day, you start making fewer mistakes and the song begins to sound more like the way you hear it in your head. After a few weeks, you not only play it without mistakes, but your piano teacher tells you it sounds terrific! In this instance, my grandfather was right: the best reward is that you can play the song the way you want to. All of your hard work paid off, and you play the song with pride for your friends and family.

In reality, some of the things people need to do not only are harder than learning a song on the piano but take longer. And the longer it takes to master a skill, the more likely it is they will lose interest and stop doing the hard work that's needed to be successful. Rewards are a way to get people to do things. For example, adults get paid when they go to work, and they appreciate it if someone gives them a bonus (eg, extra money, more vacation) because they're doing a good job.

As a pediatrician, I recommend that children get rewards in many situations. I give kids rewards (usually a piece of candy) if they have to take medicine that tastes bad. I also give kids rewards (usually a sticker) if they pee or poop on the potty when they're being toilet trained. I don't give rewards for everything. For example, I wouldn't give someone a reward for making the

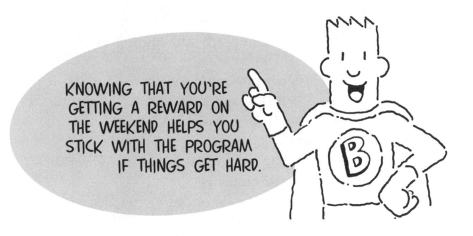

KNOWING THAT YOU'RE GETTING A REWARD ON THE WEEKEND HELPS YOU STICK WITH THE PROGRAM IF THINGS GET HARD.

bed or carrying dirty dishes to the sink. Rewards are given for situations that require extra effort.

What Types of Rewards Do I Get for Doing the Waking Up Dry Program?

Your coaches will give you a small reward once a week during the program. These rewards are for the effort you put into the program, *not* for dry nights. Once you finish the program, you will get a special reward that's like a graduation present for becoming dry.

Although rewards are an important way to recognize the effort you put into the program, don't forget that becoming dry is the best reward of all. When I see children for bedwetting visits, I ask them what they're looking forward to when they finish the program. Here are some of the answers I've received over the years. Put a ✓ by each statement that applies to you, and fill in the blank spaces if you can think of any others.

☐ I'll be able to go on sleepovers whenever I want to.

☐ I won't go to bed wondering if I'll be wet in the morning.

☐ My parents will be proud of me.

☐ I'll be proud of myself.

☐ I won't wake up in a cold, wet bed.

☐ I won't have to worry about someone finding out that I wet the bed.

☐ I'll be able to drink before bed if I want to.

☐ I won't feel like a little kid anymore.

☐ My parents won't have extra laundry to do.

☐ My room won't smell like pee.

☐ I won't have to wake up early to take care of my wet bed.

☐ I won't be embarrassed anymore.

☐ I won't have to worry that my brother or sister is going to tease me about wetting the bed.

☐ _____

☐ _____

☐ _____

☐ _____

☐ _____

☐ _____

☐ _____

☐ _____

☐ _____

☐ _____

COACH'S CORNER

I don't see why we should give our son something special just for becoming dry at night. Isn't that reward enough?

Like my grandfather, some parents think children should be motivated on their own without the need for rewards. Other parents equate rewards with bribes. On a practical level, however, they are very different. A bribe is something the child is given *before* he does what's expected of him. A reward is something the child gets *after* he carries out a task. In the former situation, the child is put in control and has the power to dawdle or refuse to hold up his end of the bargain. In the latter situation, the reward is a concrete way of saying thank you for a job well done. Despite the power of rewards, they are not an end in themselves. Rewards should always be paired with praise and encouragement. Together, they can make the difference between a cooperative and an uncooperative child. And as far as bedwetting goes, we know that rewards help.

My wife wants to give our 6-year-old a piece of candy every time she has a dry bed.

I generally don't recommend giving a child candy every time she has a dry bed. What I prefer is setting up a reward calendar on which you give your child stickers or stars every time she has a dry night. Then after she's been dry for a few days, you can, for example, give her some candy or let her pick a restaurant for dinner. I like this method because it recognizes the child's accomplishment but also lets her appreciate that she really worked for the reward.

I have a 13-year-old with primary nighttime wetting. He's very enthusiastic about the program, but he doesn't want to use a contract and doesn't care about getting weekly rewards.

continued on next page

Most children like the weekly rewards for the reasons previously described. However, if your child is motivated and has a track record of sticking with things, it's OK to do the program without these psychological extras. Remind him that the program can get difficult at times, and discuss ways you can be supportive if he gets discouraged.

CHAPTER 15

You Can Do It!

One of the things I mentioned at the beginning of the book is how important it is to practice when you're learning a new skill. When I see children in my office, I ask them if they have any heroes. Most kids answer this question by choosing a famous athlete. Others pick teachers, family members, or even famous people from the past. In each case, however, the person named is someone the child looks up to because of something that person accomplished in his or her life. For this discussion, let's say you picked a soccer player as the person you look up to. To be good at the sport, what do you think a soccer player has to do day after day? To help answer this question, I'll give you 3 choices.

1. Read about soccer.
2. Watch people play soccer.
3. Practice, practice, practice.

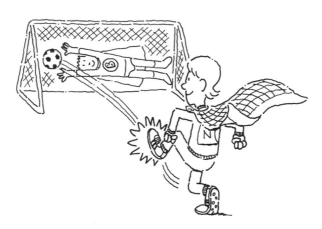

The correct answer is 3. If you want to be great at soccer, you have to practice every day. You have to practice when it's sunny outside and when it's raining outside. You have to practice when you have lots of energy and when you're tired and would rather stay home. You have to practice when you're having a great day and everything is going right and on days when you're not playing very well. This is what it takes to be really good at soccer. You also have to practice to be good at basketball, baseball, teaching, or even becoming dry at night.

There may be times during the program when you get frustrated. You might not want to do your bladder exercises. You might get up late for school and not want to fill out your calendar. If you're using the bedwetting alarm, you might have lots of wet nights in the beginning, or you might be tired from all the times you get woken up by the alarm. It's OK to be upset when this happens. Talk to your coach about it. Talk to your doctor about it. *But don't give up!* Remember what athletes have to do to be really good at something. The same thing applies to you when you're doing the Waking Up Dry Program.

There is one more thing you can do if you're discouraged about the program. Think about all the goals you have accomplished in your life. Children have to learn a million things as they grow up, and it takes lots of practice to master these skills. Here's a list of things that most kids have to work hard at to master.

• Tying your shoes
• Throwing and catching a ball
• Riding a bike
• Reading and writing
• Going across the monkey bars
• Playing a musical instrument
• Swimming
• Burping whenever you want to (just kidding)

Because each of us is different, list some of your own accomplishments in the following spaces. Ask your coaches for help if you can't think of anything right away.

- _____

- _____

- _____

- _____

- _____

Have your coaches list some of the things they have accomplished in their lives, either as adults or kids. Ask them to tell you how hard it was to accomplish these goals and the frustrations they experienced along the way.

- _____

- _____

- _____

- _____

- _____

As you get ready to start your program, remember the things you read in this chapter. If you get frustrated once you're doing the program, come back and read the chapter again. *Remember, YOU CAN DO IT!*

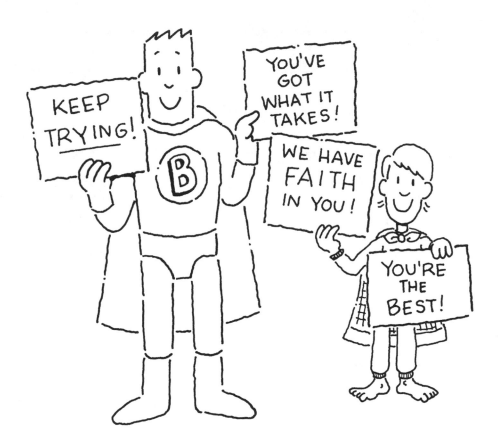

PART 4

The Bedwetting Alarm

CHAPTER 16

The Bedwetting Alarm

The purpose of the next few chapters is to introduce you to the bedwetting alarm. I will show you how to set up the program in Chapter 20.

What Is the Bedwetting Alarm?

The bedwetting alarm is a device that teaches your brain to pay attention to your bladder while you're sleeping. Bedwetting alarms have 2 basic parts: a wetness sensor that detects urine and an alarm box that buzzes after you wet the bed. Bedwetting alarms come in 3 styles: wearable alarms, wireless alarms, and bell-and-pad alarms (see Figure 16-1 on page 108).

- **Wearable alarms** are the most popular. Depending on the model you buy, the alarm box attaches to different places on your body. In most cases, you attach it to your undershirt or pajama top by the shoulder area. The sensor attaches to your underpants and connects to the alarm box with a cord.
- **Wireless alarms** use a separate alarm box that is not worn on the body. The sensor attaches to your underpants and "connects" to the alarm box with radio signals. This is similar to remote control cars that work without wires.
- **Bell-and-pad alarms** also have a sensor and an alarm box, but you don't wear anything on your body. Instead, there is a sensor pad that goes underneath your bottom sheet and an alarm box that is placed near your bed.

Figure 16-1.
Bedwetting Alarms

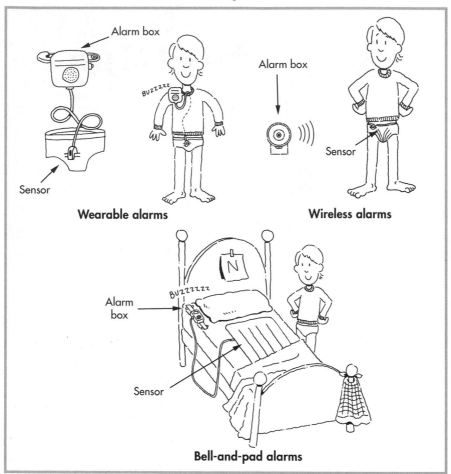

How Does the Alarm Work?

The alarm's sensor has the ability to detect small amounts of moisture. When you wet at night, the urine in your underpants turns on the alarm, creating a loud sound. When the alarm goes off, it wakes you up so you can go to the bathroom and finish peeing in the toilet. After weeks of hearing the alarm, your brain learns to pay attention to your full bladder signals and you will wake up before wetting the bed. (One of my patients told me his brain would "answer the phone" on the first ring whenever his bladder called at night.) Over time, most kids stop waking up at night to pee. This happens because your bladder learns to hold all of your urine until morning.

Newer bedwetting alarms have a light that flashes when they go off. This makes them easier to see in the dark. Some of them also have the ability to vibrate when they go off. This is a helpful feature because some kids are more likely to wake up if they feel a vibration at the same time the alarm starts to buzz.

What Do Sensors Look Like?

There are a number of bedwetting alarms currently available, and each one has its own type of sensor. The sensors used with some of the alarms are shown in Figure 16-2.

Figure 16-2.
Alarm Sensors

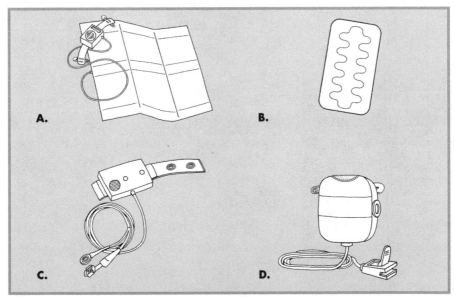

A. Sensor pad   **B.** Wireless sensor   **C.** Snap-on sensor   **D.** Clip-on sensor

How Does Urine Set Off the Alarm?

When you attach the sensor to your underpants, the metal parts are not touching each other because the fabric separates them. When you pee, urine wets your underpants and the urine allows the metal parts to "connect" with each other. When this connection is completed, the alarm goes off.

What Does *Beating the Buzzer* Mean?

When you first start using the alarm, you probably won't wake up until the alarm has gone off and your bed is wet. As you learn to respond to the alarm more quickly, you will wake up before your bladder is completely empty. *Beating the buzzer* means that you want to get up before the alarm starts to buzz or as soon as possible after it goes off. (Remember that your sphincter muscle is the muscle you use to hold in your urine.)

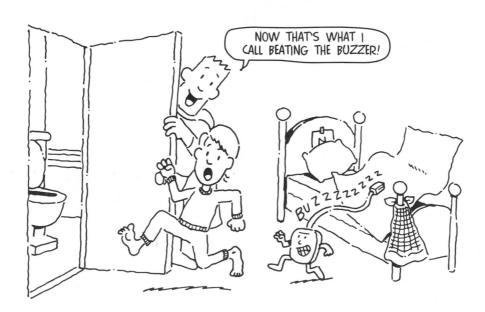

Does the Alarm Work With Children Who Are Deep Sleepers?

Bedwetting alarms are the most effective treatment for deep sleepers. However, because most kids don't wake up at the beginning of the program, it's helpful if one of your coaches sleeps in your room so you can be woken up right away. After a couple of weeks, most kids learn to respond to the alarm and your coach no longer needs to be in the room. It's still important for your coaches to be involved, however, so I recommend using a monitor (or an intercom) so they can hear the alarm if it goes off. (Some bedwetting alarms have an optional receiver that can go in the parent's bedroom.)

Does the Alarm Work Right Away?

Some kids begin having dry nights rather quickly, but most continue to wet the bed until they've been doing the program for a few weeks. Some kids become dry all of a sudden. Others continue to wet, but the size of the wet spot gets smaller and smaller until they start having dry nights. Here's a summary of what you can expect. (The time between one step and the next varies from child to child.)

1. At first, you may not hear the alarm, and you won't wake up until your coach gets you up. Your bed will be wet.

2. In a week or so, it will become easier for your coach to wake you up, but your bed will still be wet.

3. In a few weeks, you will wake up when the alarm goes off or as soon as your coach calls your name. Your bed will probably still be wet, but the size of your spots may be smaller.

4. You will begin waking up as soon as the alarm goes off, though some nights will go better than others. The bed may be wet or perhaps only your underpants will be wet.

5. You will wake up on your own every time the alarm goes off. Your underpants will be wet, but your bed will be dry.

6. You will wake up the instant the alarm goes off, and your underpants will only be damp.

7. You will wake up before you wet the bed, and your underpants will be dry.

8. Some kids will continue waking up at night to go to the bathroom.

9. Most kids will begin sleeping through the night, only now they will be completely dry.

10. It's *normal* to have setbacks along the way, meaning you may wet the bed after being dry for a week or more. As the program continues, this will happen less often, until you're completely dry. If you get frustrated, reread Chapter 15.

How Long Does It Take to Become Completely Dry?

Most children become dry within 2 months of starting the program. Some do it in a few weeks, but others aren't completely dry until they've been doing the program for 3 or 4 months.

Does the Bedwetting Alarm Work for Everyone?

If you stick with the program, your chances of becoming dry are excellent. There are a few reasons why the program doesn't work for everyone, however. Some kids lose interest if the program turns out to be harder than they expected, and this makes it more difficult to become dry. In other cases, something unexpected may occur at home that makes it harder to complete the program or do it correctly. (Remember that it's important to use your alarm *every* night.) Finally, some kids have more than one problem that's causing their wetting. If a child is a deep sleeper, has a small bladder, and wets many times a night, it takes a lot more effort to become dry. If you fall into this group, I recommend that you work on the program with your doctor because taking a medication with the alarm increases your chances for success.

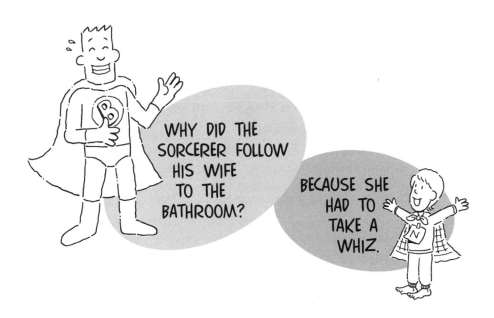

Do Kids Ever Start Wetting Again After They Become Dry?

If you start wetting again, we call it a *relapse.* Learning to be dry at night is a complicated process, and some children will have occasional wet nights for no obvious reason. Other times, kids might wet the bed because they are sick, tired, or worried about something, such as moving to a new home or starting school. Having an occasional accident is not a big deal. I discuss relapses in more detail in Chapter 25.

COACH'S CORNER

Why is it important for children to wake up quickly after the alarm goes off?

Research shows that the sooner a child wakes up after the alarm goes off, the quicker she will become dry. Most children go to sleep before their parents, so you need to be prepared to get to their rooms quickly if the alarm goes off. It's OK to use a monitor to help you do this, but stay close by, and try to get to the room as soon as possible after the alarms starts to buzz.

I have a bad back, so sleeping on the floor in my son's room will be difficult.

Although it's helpful for coaches to be nearby to ensure that their children wake up promptly, there are circumstances for which this is impractical. In addition to bad backs, a coach may not sleep well on a cot or an air mattress. In such cases, sleeping in a child's room may be a big imposition. If you can't manage this, use an intercom and make an effort to get to his room as soon as possible after the alarm goes off.

Is it possible to get a shock from the alarm?

Most bedwetting alarms are battery-operated devices that run on a very small electrical charge. I've been using these products for 35 years and have never had a patient shocked or harmed in any way.

Do bedwetting alarms require any maintenance?

Bedwetting alarms don't require much upkeep, but it's impor-tant to read the instructions that come with the device. If the battery gets low or the sensor develops a buildup of residual urine, it may cause false alarms or fail to work properly when a child wets at night. You can prevent these problems by setting off the alarm periodically and checking to see that it produces a loud sound.

Do we have to worry that the alarm's battery will die in the middle of the night?

Bedwetting alarms are unlikely to run out of power during normal use. It's possible a low battery may cause the alarm to function erratically, however. The following situations are the ones most likely to run down the battery:

- If no one wakes up and the alarm is on for an extended period of time
- If you use a vibrating model, which requires more power to work
- If your child does the program for a longer period of time or has a relapse and uses the original battery that came with the alarm

What percentage of children become dry using the bedwetting alarm?

Depending on the study one looks at, bedwetting alarms are successful 50% to 75% of the time. Programs that include other behavioral components are more effective. In my office, for example, 85% of children who use the alarm become dry within 4 months of starting the program. There are 3 things that contribute to this success.

- The program attacks bedwetting from different angles.
- I eliminate less motivated children before we start.
- I'm not dealing with a referral population, which may contain a higher percentage of children who are difficult to treat.

Approximately 15% of my patients relapse after becoming dry. Most of these children become dry if they repeat the program.

CHAPTER 17

Choosing a Bedwetting Alarm

Which alarm you should buy is a matter of personal preference. New models come out from time to time, so you can check with your doctor to see if there is a current model that will work better for you. Video demonstrations for most bedwetting alarms are available on the Internet.

Are All Alarms Created Equal?

No one has done a study comparing bedwetting alarms, but in my experience, some are better than others. The ones I like best are more acceptable to kids and are more likely to go off when you wet the bed. The following list does not include every alarm, but it provides information on models that will

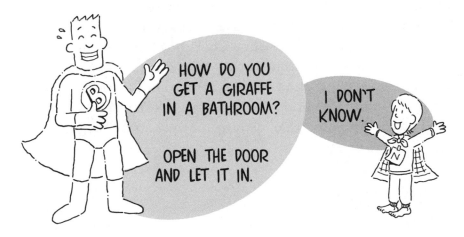

HOW DO YOU GET A GIRAFFE IN A BATHROOM?

OPEN THE DOOR AND LET IT IN.

I DON'T KNOW.

satisfy most children's needs. I use a 1 to 4 scale, with 4 stars being the best. The highest rated alarms aren't necessarily the most expensive.

Malem Wearable Alarms (★ ★ ★ ★)
$84.95 to $119.95

Malem makes a number of wearable alarms. The entry-level models produce sound without vibration. The Ultimate models come with an option for sound, sound and vibration, or vibration alone. There's even a model that lets you record your own sound or message. Malem alarms come in a variety of colors. The alarm box attaches to your shirt or pajama top with a plastic clip. (Entry-level models attach with a safety pin.) Malem alarms have a sturdy clip-on sensor that won't fall off during the night. A 2-step process turns off the alarm: first, you unhook the sensor; second, you push a button on the alarm box. This encourages you to wake up rather than turning off the alarm and going right back to sleep.

Wet-Stop3 (★ ★ ★ ½)
$50

The Wet-Stop3 is a wearable alarm that comes in 3 colors: blue, green, and pink. The alarm box attaches to your shirt or pajama top with a magnetic clasp. It can be set for sound, vibration, or both. (You can't select the sounds, but they are very loud.) It has a sturdy clip-on sensor that won't fall off during the night. A 2-step process turns off the alarm: first, you unhook the sensor; second, you push a button on the alarm box. This encourages you to wake up rather than turning off the alarm and going right back to sleep.

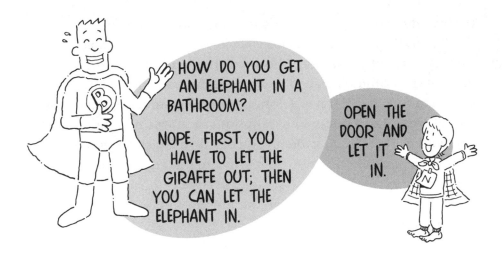

Rodger Wireless (★ ★ ★ ½)
$129.95 to $169.95

The Rodger Wireless is an alarm for kids who don't want to wear an alarm box with a cord that attaches to their underpants. Instead of using a clip-on sensor, the Rodger Wireless comes with 2 pairs of underpants that have moisture-sensitive threads sewn into the fabric. (You need to wash them before using the alarm for the first time.) The wireless transmitter attaches to the waistband with snaps. It's very sturdy and won't fall off during the night. The alarm box should be placed away from the bed so you have to get up to turn it off. It has adjustable sounds and a volume control. Two options can be used with the system: a vibrating attachment that makes it easier to wake up and an extra receiver for your parents' bedroom.

DryBuddyFLEX Wireless System (★ ★ ★ ½)
$99.99 to $158.99

The DryBuddyFLEX Wireless System is for kids who don't want to wear an alarm box with a cord that attaches to their underpants. Instead of using a clip-on sensor, the DryBuddyFLEX uses a wireless sensor that attaches to your underpants with magnets. The alarm box and the remote on/off switch should be placed away from the bed so you have to get up to turn it off. It has a volume control and a loud trumpet sound. The alarm system has 3 options: a vibrating attachment that makes it easier to wake up, an extra receiver for your parents' bedroom, and moisture-sensitive briefs that let you attach the sensor to the waistband instead of the crotch area of your underpants. (You need to wash them before using the briefs for the first time.)

Rodger Clippo (★ ★ ★ ½)
$59.95

The Rodger Clippo is a wearable alarm that attaches to your shirt or pajama top with a magnetic clasp. A switch lets you choose from 8 different sounds and a vibration mode. The front of the alarm box can be covered with stickers that come with the device. (If you buy the alarm from the Bedwetting Store, you can choose from basketball, soccer, football, and other designs.) It has a sturdy, clip-on sensor that won't fall off during the night. A 2-step process turns off the alarm: first, you unhook the sensor; second, you push a button on the alarm box. This encourages you to wake up rather than turning off the alarm and going right back to sleep.

Malem Wireless Alarm (★ ★ ★)
$139.95

The Malem Wireless Alarm is for kids who don't want to wear an alarm box by their shoulder. The alarm has a variety of sounds and a volume control, and you can buy an optional receiver for your parents' bedroom. The sensor clips to the front of your underpants, and the wireless transmitter hooks to the waistband of your underpants. It's bulkier than the Rodger Wireless and DryBuddyFLEX alarms.

Malem Bedside Alarm (★ ★ ★)
$169.95

I don't recommend bell-and-pad models often, but the Malem Bedside Alarm is for kids who don't want to wear anything on their bedclothes. The alarm has 8 random sounds and a volume control. You can buy an optional vibratory unit and a wireless receiver for your parents' bedroom.

Chummie (★ ★ ½)
$99.99

The Chummie is a wearable alarm that produces a loud chirping sound and vibration when it goes off. The sensor is made of flexible material that's attached to the outside of your underpants with metallic tape that comes with the device. (The sensor does not stay attached unless it's sandwiched between 2 pairs of underpants.) Removing the sensor cord and pushing a button on the alarm box turn it off. Only one step is required to turn off the alarm, so kids may fall back asleep before their coaches know the alarm went off. The plastic clip that attaches the alarm box to your shirt or pajama top has a tendency to pop off when kids try to put it on.

Nytone (★ ★ ½)
$89.99

The Nytone is a wearable alarm that produces a beeping sound and vibration when it goes off. Instead of attaching to your shoulder area, the Nytone is worn on the upper arm with an adjustable band. Wearing the alarm on the upper arm will be a disadvantage for some kids, but others may prefer wearing it there instead of by the shoulder. The cord attaches to your underpants with a clip-on sensor. You turn the alarm off by pulling the cord from the alarm box. Only one step is required to turn off the alarm, so kids may fall back asleep before their coaches know the alarm went off.

SleepDry (★ ★)
$53.95

The SleepDry is a wearable alarm that produces a loud buzz. The alarm box attaches to your shirt or pajama top with metal snaps. The sensor consists of metal snaps that attach to your underpants. The snaps don't touch your skin because you wear 2 pairs of underpants to bed, and the snaps attach to the outside pair. You turn the alarm off by pulling the snaps apart. Although they are easy to use, the snaps loosen up over time and can come undone during the night. Only one step is required to turn off the alarm, so kids may fall back asleep before their coaches know the alarm went off.

DRI Excel (★ ★)
$69.95

The DRI Excel is a wearable alarm that produces a loud chirping sound when it goes off. The sensor is made of flexible material that's designed to be placed inside 2 pairs of underpants or inside a panty liner. (It won't stay in place unless you use a panty liner.) Unplugging the sensor cord from the alarm box turns it off. Only one step is required to turn off the alarm, so kids may fall back asleep before their coaches know the alarm went off.

Night Hawk (★ ½)
$156

The Night Hawk alarm consists of a small box that's worn inside the fly area of boy's briefs or between 2 pairs of girl's panties. The alarm can be set for sound and vibration or vibration alone. The alarm is kept in place with a plastic clip but has a number of drawbacks. Some children won't like wearing a vibrating alarm in their underpants. It doesn't go off consistently in response to wetting episodes. Only one step is required to turn off the alarm, so kids may fall back asleep before their coaches know the alarm went off.

COACH'S CORNER

What are the most important features to look for when we purchase a bedwetting alarm?

When I see children in my office, I show them display models for the alarms mentioned in this chapter.

Although I let them play a role in which model they choose, I have my own bias based on how well the alarms work. The most important thing is to pick a comfortable model that's reliable. A reliable alarm stays attached at night, encourages the child to wake up to turn it off, and buzzes when it's supposed to. In addition, because most children don't wake up by themselves at the beginning of the program, you need an alarm that buzzes (with or without vibration) so you'll be alerted when it goes off.

Where can we buy bedwetting alarms?

Bedwetting alarms can be purchased directly from the manufacturer and from resellers such as the Bedwetting Store and Amazon.com. The Wet-Stop3 is manufactured and sold by

continued on next page

PottyMD. Malem and Rodger alarms are made in Europe and can be purchased from the Bedwetting Store and Amazon.com.

Insurance companies sometimes reimburse patients for the cost of bedwetting alarms. How much they pay depends on your deductible and the type of insurance you have. It may help to get a prescription from your doctor that says "medical device" before filing a claim.

CHAPTER 18

Getting Familiar With Your Alarm

Before you use your bedwetting alarm, you should become familiar with its parts. It may be easier to practice attaching and unhooking the sensor if you use a pair of underpants that you're not wearing. After you do this a few times, wet the sensor with water to make the alarm buzz. Listen to the sound for a few moments. Then turn it off. Once you're able to connect the alarm and turn it off easily, practice again, only this time attach it to the underpants you're wearing. Wet the sensor again to see what it will be like when the alarm goes off for real.

When I teach children how to use the alarm in my office, they are usually fascinated with the sound and the way the sensor turns the alarm off and on. I hear from parents that kids often play with their alarms when they get them home. Although this is perfectly normal, keep in mind that pets, small children, and some adults are sensitive to loud sounds. Therefore, it's a good idea if you don't go overboard with this goofing around.

Before you use your alarm for the first time, you should have a practice session with your coach to rehearse what will happen at night. On the first practice run, I want you to pretend you're too sleepy to wake up. This will give your coach a chance to try the wake-up drill. It will also let you see what coaches have to go through sometimes to wake their kids up at night. The

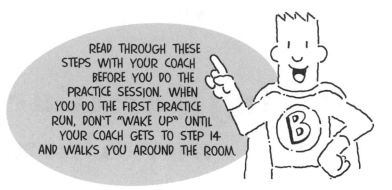

READ THROUGH THESE STEPS WITH YOUR COACH BEFORE YOU DO THE PRACTICE SESSION. WHEN YOU DO THE FIRST PRACTICE RUN, DON'T "WAKE UP" UNTIL YOUR COACH GETS TO STEP 14 AND WALKS YOU AROUND THE ROOM.

alarm must continue to buzz until you "wake up" and turn it off yourself. On the second practice run, I want you to get up quickly so you can *beat the buzzer.* Waking up quickly and beating the buzzer are what you should shoot for every night.

Supplies You'll Need at Home

• A bedwetting alarm
• A wet washcloth

First Practice Run

1. Attach the alarm unit to your undershirt or other location.

2. Attach the sensor to your underpants.

3. Lie down and pretend you're asleep.

4. Your coach will drip some water on your underpants to set off the alarm.

5. When the alarm goes off, pretend you're still asleep.

6. Your coach will call your name and say the wake-up message: "Timmy, you need to wake up! Wake up, Timmy! Timmy, you can do it! You need to wake up and beat the buzzer if you want to have dry beds." (**Coach's Tip:** Your tone should be animated and encouraging.)

7. Don't wake up yet.

8. Your coach will gently shake your shoulders 3 or 4 times and repeat the wake-up message.

9. Pretend you're still asleep.

10. Your coach will sit you up in bed and repeat the wake-up message.

11. Boy, are you sleepy! Don't wake up yet.

12. Your coach will wet your face 2 or 3 times with a washcloth and repeat the wake-up message.

13. You're a real zombie tonight! Don't wake up yet.

14. Your coach will repeat the wake-up message and walk you around the room. (Don't make it hard for your coach to get you out of bed.)

15. Now you can wake up.

16. Turn off the alarm, and go to the bathroom like you will if your alarm goes off in the middle of the night.

17. Come back to your room, change your underpants, and reconnect your alarm.

Second Practice Run

1. The second session should proceed just like the first, except this time I want you to get up as soon as your coach calls your name.

2. Turn off the alarm, and go to the bathroom like you will in the middle of the night.

3. Come back to your room, change your underpants, and reconnect your alarm.

Waking Up at Night

When you do the program for real, it helps if you're fully awake once the alarm goes off because you're more likely to cooperate with your coaches if you are alert when you get up at night. This should go smoothly most of the time. On some nights, however, the alarm may go off when you're in such a deep sleep that a fire engine wouldn't wake you up (see Your Child Is Sleepy or Grumpy When He Wakes Up on page 178).

FUN FACT Have you ever noticed your urine smells funny after you eat asparagus? (Wait, kids eat asparagus?!) This happens because asparagus has a chemical in it that creates a particular smell when it comes out in the urine. What's really interesting, however, is that some people don't know about this odor because the smell center in their brain doesn't recognize it. If you tell these people about "asparagus pee," they will think you're nuts! Now you can enlighten them.

Tips for Hooking Up Your Alarm

The way you attach the alarm depends on which one you buy. Each alarm comes with its own instructions, and you should follow these guidelines carefully. However, I have learned a number of tips over the years that apply to most alarms.

• The cord that attaches to your underpants is supposed to go inside your shirt or pajama top. If you don't like the way this feels, wear 2 shirts to bed and run the cord between them. If this makes you too hot, wear 1 shirt and secure the cord to the outside of your shirt with a small clip or masking tape.

• If the cord is too long, secure it to your shirt with a small clip or masking tape.

- Even though bedwetting alarms are light, they bother some kids because they occasionally make shirts sag. If this happens to you, wear tighter-fitting shirts or attach the alarm box closer to your shoulder area.
- Boys should attach the sensor to the front of their underpants, and girls should attach it to the bottom of their underpants. This is important because you want the alarm to go off as soon as possible and urine comes out of boys in the front and girls between the legs.
- It's important that clip-on or snap-on sensors fit snugly, or they may come undone during the night.
- Bedwetting alarms work best if they go off right after you pee. Therefore, you should always sleep in snug-fitting underpants instead of boxer-type underpants or pajama bottoms.
- Alarms that attach to shirts with metal snaps will damage fabric over time. Therefore, don't wear the alarm with your favorite clothes. Alarms that attach to shirts with safety pins can stick your skin, so be careful when you put them on.
- Children sometimes don't like the way sensors feel in their underwear. If you can't get used to this after a few days, wear a second pair of underpants inside the pair with the sensor.
- Girls should not wear nightgowns to bed because this makes it harder to turn off the alarm.
- If you don't like the idea of wearing an alarm on your upper body, consider a wireless model or one of the bell-and-pad alarms discussed in Chapter 17.

CHAPTER 19

Using Your Alarm

The purpose of this chapter is to review everything you need to do to use your bedwetting alarm. Using the alarm may seem complicated at first, but after a couple of nights, you'll be handling it like a pro! And don't forget, your coach will be there to help you.

Because you will be woken up by the alarm (or your coach), I recommend that you start the program on a Friday or Saturday night. That way, you don't have to worry about getting up for school while you're adjusting to the program. If you sleep in a bunk bed, make sure you use the bottom bed. Finally, it's a good idea to finish all of your nighttime activities before you put on your alarm.

Getting Ready for Bed

1. Get ready for bed the way you normally do. Change into your pajamas or nighttime underpants, and brush your teeth.

2. Take out 2 extra sets of underpants, pajamas, sheets, and blankets before going to sleep so you don't have to hunt for them in the middle of the night. If you use disposable underpads, take out 2 of them as well (see Chapter 26).

3. If you wet the bed, you'll need a place to put your wet underpants and bedding. Most kids put this stuff in their bathroom. If you don't want your brothers or sisters to see your wet sheets, pick another spot. One option is to use a laundry basket or plastic pail that's kept in your coach's bathroom. Don't keep wet bedding in your bedroom because that will make the room smell like urine.

4. Turn on your night-light or another light so your room isn't completely dark. It helps if the hallway has a night-light in it as well.

5. Put on your bedwetting alarm.

6. Do your waking up practice.

7. Remind yourself that you are the boss of your bladder and you are going to wake up quickly if you can't hold all of your urine until morning.

KID'S ALERT See the Keeping Disposable Underpads in Place section on page 197 for a tip that makes it easier to deal with wet beds in the middle of the night.

What to Do When the Alarm Goes Off

1. If your alarm goes off, you need to wake up right away and beat the buzzer. This means you should squeeze your sphincter muscle quickly to hold back any urine that's still in your bladder.

2. If you don't wake up when the alarm goes off, your coach will do the wake-up drill to get you up.

3. Turn off your alarm as soon as you wake up. If you have trouble turning off the alarm, your coach can help, but you should be the one to turn it off.

4. Go to the bathroom and finish peeing in the toilet. If your bladder is empty, that's OK. You'll try to beat the buzzer tomorrow night.

5. Come back to your room, and change into dry clothes.

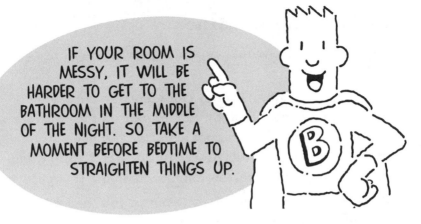

IF YOUR ROOM IS MESSY, IT WILL BE HARDER TO GET TO THE BATHROOM IN THE MIDDLE OF THE NIGHT. SO TAKE A MOMENT BEFORE BEDTIME TO STRAIGHTEN THINGS UP.

6. If possible, help your coach remove the wet bedding and re-make the bed. If you are too tired, your coach will do it for you.

7. Reconnect your bedwetting alarm.

8. Turn off your regular light, and get into bed.

9. Feel your sheets and imagine waking up in a nice dry bed.

10. Remind yourself that you are the boss of your bladder and you are going to wake up if you can't hold all of your urine until morning.

Alice's Story

Alice is a 10-year-old who wet the bed about 4 nights a week. She did not want her little brother to know about her wetting because it bothered her that she was wet at night and he wasn't. After talking with Alice about her concern, we came up with the following solution: Alice's mom gave her and her brother some chores to do around the house. Her brother's chore was to set and clear the table at dinner. Alice's chore was to take the dirty clothes to the laundry room in the morning. Whenever she had an accident, Alice put her wet bedding in with the other clothes and carried the laundry basket to the basement. Alice was very proud of her ability to take care of this problem on her own.

Your Morning Routine

What you do in the morning depends on whether or not you had a dry night.

1. Fill out your Waking Up Dry calendar to record what happened during the night. *Remember that your coaches need to agree with you about whether you had a dry or wet night.* (See the Kid's Alert box on page 55 and Chapter 25 on page 181 for a few comments about this process.)

2. If you had a dry night, put a sticker on your calendar or record *D* for *dry* in the space. If your underpants were wet but your bedding was dry, record *SW* for *small wet* on your calendar. If your underpants and bedding were wet, record *LW* for *large wet* on your calendar.

3. If you had a dry night, feel your sheets and think about how great it's going to be to have dry beds every night.

4. If you had a wet night, review what happened during the night and give yourself a thumbs-up for cooperating with the program.

5. Put your alarm and calendar in a drawer or other safe place so no one will find them by accident.

6. Get dressed and go to breakfast.

7. Remind yourself to do your bladder exercises during the day.

Keep Your Alarm From Breaking

It's easy for bedwetting alarms to end up in laundry baskets attached to your bedclothes. This is especially true for the sensors that come with wireless models. An alarm or sensor that's gone through the wash will no longer work, and this type of damage is not covered by the device's warranty. One way to prevent this from happening is to have one of your coaches put a note on the washing machine that says, "Check for alarm."

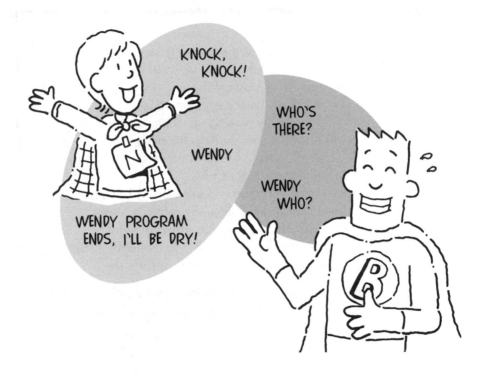

COACH'S CORNER

Do you have any final suggestions about the bedwetting alarm?

Here are a few tips to keep in mind before you start the program.

- Most children do not wake up when the alarm buzzes at the beginning of the program.

Therefore, it's important you're close by when it goes off. Because you obviously can't sit in your child's room until you go to sleep, put a monitor in the room and be ready to get there quickly if the alarm buzzes. Most children wet the bed within a few hours of going to sleep.

continued on next page

- Until your child demonstrates the ability to wake up when the alarm goes off, it's helpful if you sleep in his room so you can wake him up. In most cases, you will only have to do this for a week or so, but it's time well spent.
- Once your child is reliably waking up at night, you don't need to rush to his room immediately. It's still important that you get up, however, because most children need help (or supervision) after the alarm goes off.
- The most common reason alarms don't work is because people use them incorrectly. Follow the manufacturer's instructions carefully, and use the alarm *every* night.
- When you review what happened during the night, praise your child for his cooperation with the program.

My son doesn't want to help with his bedding if he wets the bed at night. Isn't this his responsibility?

It's OK to encourage kids to help out if they wet the bed at night, but they should *never* be forced to do this. Children are usually very tired when the alarm wakes them up (as are adults), and having to deal with a wet bed may sour their attitude toward the entire program. Try breaking down the process into smaller steps. For example, your son may be willing to remove his underpad or top sheet. This allows him to take some responsibility for cleaning up but isn't as taxing as remaking the entire bed. And don't forget the tips in Chapter 26 that make it easier to deal with wet beds in the middle of the night.

PART 5

Putting the Program Together

CHAPTER 20

Setting Up the Program

When I work with kids in my office, we set up their programs at our second visit. Although some parts are important for everyone, I let them fine-tune the program if they want to. (*Fine-tuning the program* means you get to make some decisions about what you do.) Let's review each part of the program so you can set it up to fit your needs.

- **The Waking Up Dry calendar** is important for everyone. Fill out your calendar every morning as discussed in the Your Morning Routine section on page 134. Don't forget to put a check on your calendar if you wake up on your own when the alarm goes off.
- **Waking up practice** is important for everyone. Do waking up practice every night.
- **The bedwetting alarm** is the main part of the program. It's obviously important for everyone.
- **Bladder exercises** such as water gulping is what I usually recommend at the beginning of the program. (Remember that you can skip this step if you already drink a lot during the day.) Although most children prefer this exercise as well, some kids don't like having to drink extra water during the day. Either it's too hard to remember, it interferes with their appetite, or they don't want to use the bathroom at school.

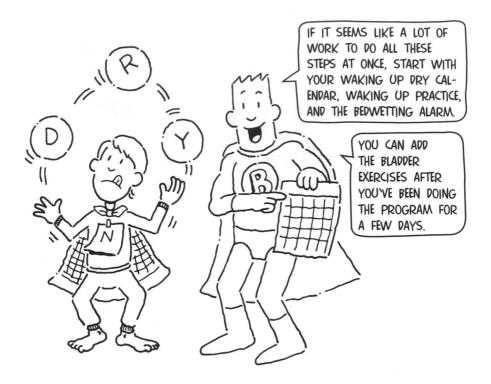

IF IT SEEMS LIKE A LOT OF WORK TO DO ALL THESE STEPS AT ONCE, START WITH YOUR WAKING UP DRY CALENDAR, WAKING UP PRACTICE, AND THE BEDWETTING ALARM.

YOU CAN ADD THE BLADDER EXERCISES AFTER YOU'VE BEEN DOING THE PROGRAM FOR A FEW DAYS.

(See the Coach's Corner box on page 93 for some tips on how you can make water gulping easier to do.) If it's too hard to do water gulping, you can do the bladder attention exercise instead.

- The **Waking Up Dry contract** is the part of the program kids love the most because using the contract lets you earn your weekly and special rewards (see Chapter 21).

Finishing the Program

I mentioned earlier that I consider bedwetting to be "cured" when you've been dry for 14 nights in a row. Experience has taught me, however, that stopping the program right away increases your chances of having a relapse. (A *relapse* is when you start wetting the bed after you've been dry for a while.)

Therefore, I suggest a "cooling down" period during which you stop the program gradually.

1. After you've been dry for 14 nights in a row, wear the alarm every other night for 2 more weeks. On the nights when you're not wearing the alarm, leave it on your night table so you can see it before you go to sleep. If you don't have a night table, put the alarm on a chair next to your bed. Remind yourself that you are the boss of your body and you will wake up at night if you need to pee.

2. While you're wearing the alarm every other night, you can stop doing your bladder exercises and waking up practice, but you should continue to use your calendar.

3. If you're dry every night during this 2-week period, the program is finished and it's time to get your special reward (see Chapter 21).

4. If you wet the bed during this 2-week period, restart the program.

5. When you've been dry for another 14 nights in a row, go back to Step 1 and repeat the "cooling down" period.

6. If you start wetting again, ask your coach about adding a technique called *overlearning* to the program (see the Dealing With Relapses section on pages 188–189).

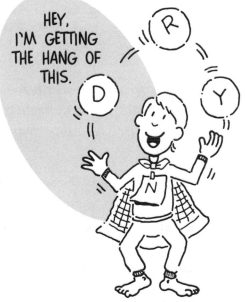

COACH'S CORNER

My wife and I are getting ready to start the program with our daughter. Does one of us have to do everything?

Parents often ask how they should divide up their coaching responsibilities. There are lots of ways to work this out, though in most cases one parent acts as the head coach and the other parent helps out as needed. (The time when head coaches need the most help is when alarms go off in the middle of the night.) If there are 2 head coaches, you can alternate responsibilities from day to day.

My son has attention-deficit/hyperactivity disorder (ADHD), and I'm concerned he won't be able to follow all the steps in your program.

If children have ADHD, learning disabilities, or certain psychological problems, the program may overwhelm them. When I run into this situation at work, I make things as easy as possible. One way to accomplish this is to concentrate on the bedwetting alarm and not bother with bladder exercises or waking up practice. (I still recommend the calendar and contract.) If the child isn't making progress by the time he's 3 to 4 weeks into the program, I consider adding these other elements at that time.

My 7-year-old doesn't have ADHD, but I still think the program is too complicated for her.

Although I generally simplify the program only for the situations previously noted, you can choose this option if you think the full program will be too much for your child. You can also simplify the program if your child becomes exhausted from being woken up by the alarm.

I bought your book for my 9-year-old son, but he doesn't want to read it.

Sometimes children have an approach/avoidance reaction when it comes to working on medical problems. If your son hasn't treated his bedwetting in the past, he may need a little time to get used to the idea. Give him a week to think about it. Then talk to him again.

If your son tried to become dry in the past and failed, it's natural he'd react this way. This occurs because some people, especially children, find it safer to accept a problem than to risk failing again. The best thing to do is to leave the book in a non-public spot in your home. Tell your son he can look at the book if he wants to, but make it clear that it's up to him. I would also tell him that looking at the book does not mean he has to do the program. Let him know you're available to discuss the situation any time he wants to. There's a reasonable chance his interest may grow in a few weeks if you don't push the issue.

My 11-year-old wets the bed almost every night. One of my friends recently suggested we take him to a specialist.

In most cases, your regular doctor will be able to treat your child's wetting. However, if you're not getting the help you need in this setting, there are 2 specialists who have an interest in bedwetting. Pediatric urologists are surgeons who specialize in the urinary tract. They're experts in bedwetting and spend a lot of their time helping children become dry. Urologists are particularly skilled in helping children with complicated types of wetting. Pediatric nephrologists are pediatricians that specialize in kidney problems. They also know a lot about wetting problems.

One thing to keep in mind is that while urologists and nephrologists are very knowledgeable about bedwetting, some of them are more inclined to use medication than behavioral techniques with children. If you see a specialist, discuss the pros and cons of each approach so you can choose the one that's best for your child.

We recently bought your book for our 13-year-old. He is very interested in the bedwetting alarm, but he wants to do it without our help.

I'm always pleased when children are motivated to become dry, but the program is too complicated for a 13-year-old to do on

continued on next page

his own. The first question to ask is why your son wants to do the program by himself. Because children are often embarrassed by their bedwetting, it's possible that doing it by himself will give your son a degree of privacy that improves his self-esteem. It's also possible that an adolescent who's working on his independence merely wants to do things without his parent's involvement.

Have a discussion with your son so you can understand his reasoning. What you should tell him, however, is that the program is more likely to succeed if he has adult supervision. Therefore, if your son refuses to do the program with you, ask him to enlist the help of his doctor. That way, you can take on a supportive role, and he can have some of the independence he is seeking.

Do you have any final suggestions before families begin the program?

- Try to remain enthusiastic and encouraging as your child goes through the program.
- Praise your child for all of her accomplishments with the program, not just dry nights.
- Be sympathetic if your child gets discouraged. Listen first. Then make suggestions. If possible, try to come up with solutions together.
- *Never* hold back weekly rewards because your child misbehaved in some other part of her life.
- Give your child help when she needs it, but let her take the lead whenever possible. Remind her this is her program and she is the star of the show.
- If your child needs stickers for her calendar or some other attention concerning the program, stop what you're doing right away to demonstrate your interest in the program.
- Use gentle reminders if your child forgets to do parts of the program so she doesn't misinterpret your help as nagging.
- Finally, if you're feeling exhausted as you go through the program, remember this line by comedy writer Gene Perret: "Parenting requires patience, endurance, forgiveness, and understanding. And if the children aren't willing to do that, it's going to be tough."

CHAPTER 21

Waking Up Dry Contract

The purpose of this chapter is to help you set up you own personal contract for the Waking Up Dry Program. Before we get to the contract, however, I want you to make some decisions about the rewards you'll get for doing the program.

Weekly Rewards

Here are some examples of the weekly rewards I recommend for the program. These are just examples, so feel free to come up with your own ideas. As a general rule, these rewards should take place on the weekend so they don't interfere with school or work schedules.

• Take a friend to the movies.

• Have a special outing with one of your coaches.

• Get an extra hour of TV or computer time.

• Do a special art project with one of your coaches.

• Go out for a special dessert.

• Get a small item such as a pack of baseball cards.

You and your coaches must agree to the specific choices you make for these rewards. For example, if your parents don't allow you to watch certain types of movies, you can't choose them as rewards for the program. On the other hand, if you want to watch the same movie 3 weeks in a row, your coaches should agree to that request.

My choices for weekly rewards are

* _____

* _____

* _____

* _____

* _____

* _____

Special Rewards

Here are some examples of special rewards you can choose
for completing the program.

* A medium-sized toy, such as a Lego set or doll
* A sleeping bag
* A stuffed animal
* A dress or jacket
* A computer game or toy
* A piece of sports equipment, such as a tennis racket,
  basketball, or hockey stick

As with the weekly rewards, you and your coaches must
agree to the specific choice you make for your special reward.
For example, if your parents don't allow you to play with certain types of toys, you can't choose one of them as a reward
for the program.

My special reward for completing the program is

* _____

Waking Up Dry Contract

1. I will begin my Waking Up Dry Program on _____ (date).

    My coaches for the program are _____

    _____.

    I agree to cooperate with my coaches until the program
    is done.

2. In addition to using the bedwetting alarm, I agree to add
    the following helper treatments to the program (check all
    that apply):
    ☐ Waking Up Dry calendar
    ☐ Water gulping
    ☐ Bladder attention
    ☐ Waking up practice

3. I understand that being tired can make it harder to stay dry
    at night, so I agree to go to bed at a reasonable hour. On
    school nights, I will go to bed at _____ pm. On nonschool
    nights, I will go to bed at _____ pm.

4. Although my bedwetting is "cured" when I have had 14 dry
    nights in a row, the program is not finished until I complete
    the "cooling down" period described in Chapter 20.

5. I know it takes practice to become dry and the program
    may last 3 to 4 months. I also know if I stick with the
    program, my chances of becoming dry are excellent.

6. I understand that my coaches are here to help me. They
    will read the book to me if I need assistance, and they will
    review the book with me as I do the program. Although my
    coaches will encourage and guide me, they promise not
    to nag. If we disagree about any part of the program, we
    will review the book together to figure out the best way to
    do things.

7. Because it takes work to become dry at night, my coaches will give me a reward once a week during the program. These rewards are for the effort I put into the program, *not* for dry nights. My coaches and I will choose these rewards before the program begins. In addition, I will get a special reward after I have completed the "cooling down" period and the program is finished. My coaches and I will agree to this reward before the program starts.

8. If the program turns out to be harder than I expected, my coaches will encourage me to continue. They will do this by continuing to praise me for all the work I've done and reminding me of the progress I've made. My coaches will not force me to complete the program if I choose to quit. If I decide to do the program in the future, they will be there to help and support me.

_____ (date)

_____ (your signature)

_____ (coach's signature)

_____ (coach's signature)

WHAT DO YOU WANT FOR YOUR SPECIAL REWARD?

SOUNDS GOOD TO ME.

AN INTERGALACTIC PLUTONIUM-POWERED SPACE SCOOTER.

PART 6

Extra Stuff for Kids

CHAPTER 22

Sleepovers

Children often ask me what they should do about sleepovers. The answer to this question depends on several factors.

- Is the sleepover happening before or after you start the program?
- Do people outside the family know you wet the bed?
- Do you want to go on sleepovers?
- Would you prefer not going on sleepovers?

One of the things I've noticed over the years is that children sleep away from home at a much earlier age than in the past. When I was a child, my friends and I didn't have sleepovers until we were 10 or 11 years old. Nowadays, kids sleep at their friend's homes when they are as young as 5 or 6. Because bed-wetting improves as children get older, going on sleepovers at a younger age means more kids have to decide how they are going to handle these events.

Sleepovers begin when children ask their friends to stay over on Friday or Saturday nights. In time, kids start having slumber parties at which as many as 10 friends sleep over at a time. The next type of outing children may be invited to is a camping trip. Camping trips begin as 1- or 2-night events with a friend's family. As kids get older, they attend summer camps that may end with overnight trips. Children also attend sleep-away camps that typically range from 1 to 4 weeks away from home. For the purposes of this discussion, all of these events can be grouped together under the heading *overnights*.

When Is the Overnight Taking Place?

Most likely you have already made some decisions about sleeping away from home. As you read this chapter, you can decide whether or not what you've been doing works for you or you'd like to consider some other options. If you haven't gone on any overnights, consider finishing the program before sleeping away from home. Once you become dry, your confidence will go up and your first overnight should be a great success! Don't skip this chapter, however, because it will help you decide what to do about overnights.

Do People Outside the Family Know That You Wet the Bed?

Whether or not people outside the family know about your wetting is an important question because it lies at the heart of how you should approach overnights. If you're not worried about having a wet night at a friend's house, everything else is easy.

Some people think you should be open about your bedwetting. They believe that keeping it a secret adds to your embarrassment and that taking a matter-of-fact attitude can reduce these feelings. Most doctors take the opposite position; they worry you might be teased if other people find out about your wetting. The decision is yours. If you decide not to talk about your wetting outside the family, there is *no reason* for you to be ashamed about it. Always remember that bedwetting is a medical condition.

What to Do if You Don't Want to Go on Overnights

Do you remember how I mentioned in Chapter 1 that you're not the only one who wets the bed? I gave you this information not only to make you feel better but also because it helps you understand the facts. Well, guess what? Kids who wet at night are not the only ones who avoid sleepovers. As a doctor, I can confidently say this topic comes up with other patients as well. Here are some situations in which kids may prefer to sleep at home.

- **Eczema (EGG-ze-ma)** is a condition that gives kids rashes on their skin. Children with eczema need to put medicine on their skin before going to bed, and they may not want their friends to see them when they have a rash or are covered with cream.
- **Sleepwalking** is a condition in which kids get up at night and walk around in a dreamlike state. They generally don't fall or get hurt, but it might be embarrassing to do this at a friend's house, and it could be dangerous in an unfamiliar setting.
- **Thumb-sucking** usually stops by the time a child turns 6 years old. However some kids don't break the habit until they're older, and they may put their thumb in their mouth unintentionally after they fall asleep. If someone sees this, it could be very embarrassing.
- **Fear of the dark is normal for children.** However, being afraid of the dark can make going on sleepovers too scary.
- **Anxiety** about leaving home can be overwhelming. Some kids don't like to be away from home. Either they miss their parents or they're just anxious (worried) when they are away. For these children, going on overnights causes a lot of distress.

If someone asks you to go on an overnight, you should have an answer ready so it won't look like you're fumbling around for an excuse. This is a great time to talk to your coach. My favorite response is simple and direct: "I'd like to come, but my parents don't let me go on sleepovers." If your friend asks why they don't let you go, use either of the following responses:

- "When I go on sleepovers, I stay up late, which makes me very grumpy the next day."
- "I've got plans tomorrow, and my parents told me I need to get a good night's sleep."

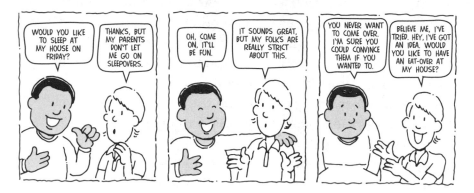

In my experience, both responses work pretty well, and your friends should drop the matter quickly. If the invitation is for a slumber party, you can go to the party, but leave late in the evening before the other kids go to bed. For this to work, your parents should talk to your friend's mom or dad to find out when everyone is expected to go to sleep. That way, your parents can pick you up as late as possible so you don't miss much. Your parents might even be able to bring you back in the morning so you can have breakfast with everyone.

There is one more thing you can do to feel connected with your friends even though you don't go on overnights; invite some kids to your house for eat-overs. These can be get-togethers where you have a few friends come over for a special kid-friendly meal. Here are some ideas.

- A backward meal where you eat dessert first and food last
- A meal where you eat everything with your fingers

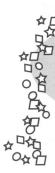

FUN FACT People with diabetes have extra sugar in their urine. It the old days, doctors had to taste their patient's urine to make this diagnosis. Nowadays, we have machines that can do this for us. Thank heavens!

- A breakfast where everyone comes in his or her pajamas
- A "dog" meal where you eat everything without using your hands

Talk with your coach and see if you can come up with some other good ideas and list them here.

- _____

- _____

- _____

What to Do if You Want to Go on Overnights

As I mentioned earlier, if you don't keep your bedwetting a secret, going on overnights is easy. Your parents should talk to your friend's mom or dad before the overnight so they know about your wetting. When you go on the overnight, you can use Pull-Ups to get a good night's sleep and make your morning routine easier.

If you decide to keep your bedwetting a secret, going on overnights is trickier, but you can definitely make it work.

Tips That Work for Any Type of Overnight

- Try the medicine desmopressin before the overnight (see Chapter 27). If this keeps you consistently dry, you won't need to do anything else to make overnights a success.
- Get a good night's sleep the night before you go away.
- Try not to eat late into the evening, and reduce your intake of liquids after dinner. This is different from my day-to-day advice (see page 170), but it makes sense to be extra careful when you sleep away from home. If possible, avoid salty food or drinks with caffeine that will increase the amount of urine you make at night.
- Make sure you pee right before you go to sleep. When you're in the bathroom, take your time and empty your bladder completely.
- Kids usually bring sleeping bags to overnights. Place your sleeping bag where it will cause the least amount of distraction if you have to get up in the middle of the night to use the bathroom.
- If you use Pull-Ups, bring one for every night you'll be away, plus one extra in case something goes wrong. (I've heard stories where the elastic band breaks, making the Pull-Up unusable.)
- Bring a sealable plastic bag for each Pull-Up you plan to use.
- Consider telling a parent or camp counselor about your wetting in case you need some help during the night or in the morning after you wake up.

DR B IS USING THE WORD PULL-UP IN A GENERAL WAY. LOTS OF KIDS ARE TOO BIG FOR PULL-UPS. THEY CAN BUY OTHER BRANDS SUCH AS UNDERJAMS TO GET THE JOB DONE.

Nathaniel's and Keisha's Stories

Although I generally advise my patients not to tell anyone about their bedwetting, I occasionally hear stories about children who don't keep it a secret.

- Nathaniel is a 7-year-old who went to a slumber party with one of my patients. There were 6 kids at the party, and when they got ready for bed, Nathaniel said to everyone, "I wear Pull-Ups at night, and I don't want anyone to tease me about it." Nathaniel was not timid or embarrassed when he said this to the other kids. No one teased him at the party or at school in the weeks that followed.

- A few years ago, I saw an 8-year-old for a bedwetting visit. When I asked Keisha if she kept her bedwetting a secret, she told me the only person outside the family who knew about it was her best friend Vanessa. When Keisha was 7, she and her mom discussed whether or not it would be a good idea to tell anyone about her bedwetting. Keisha's mom was worried that kids might tease her if they found out about it. Then Keisha's mom had an idea. She realized that telling one person didn't mean they had to tell everyone. So Keisha's mom called Vanessa's mom and asked her if she thought it would be a good idea if the girls had a "secret telling" visit at which each girl shared a special secret with the other. Vanessa's mom loved the idea because Vanessa sucked her thumb at night and was afraid to go on sleepovers. So the girls went to lunch with their moms and afterward told each other their special secrets. The experience proved to be wonderful for both of them. They had sleepovers with each other after that and felt a special bond because each one knew something personal about the other.

How to Use a Pull-Up in a Sleeping Bag

Children sleep in a variety of bedclothes at night—underpants, pajamas, nightgowns, and extra-long T-shirts. In the warmer months, children sometimes sleep in the same shorts they wore during the day. Whatever you decide to sleep in, choose clothing that fits loosely because it will hide your Pull-Up in case you need to get up at night. For boys, boxers hide Pull-Ups better than snug-fitting underpants. For girls, baggy pajama shorts or nightgowns do the job nicely.

There are many ways that you can use a Pull-Up in a sleeping bag. The following method works best if you have a place to change before you go to sleep:

1. Before you leave home, put a Pull-Up inside your shorts or boxers and place them at the bottom of your overnight bag. Put a sealable plastic bag in your overnight bag as well.

2. When you get ready for bed, put on the Pull-Up when you go to the bathroom to brush your teeth.

3. Get into your sleeping bag as soon as you put on the Pull-Up. (If you goof around with your friends, someone may notice what you're wearing.)

4. Consider having an adult wake you up around 6:00 or 7:00 am so you can take care of the Pull-Up before the other kids wake up.

KID'S ALERT If you plan to sleep in a bed instead of a sleeping bag, put on the Pull-Up using the method just described.

5. When you get up in the morning, take your overnight bag to the bathroom with you. Remove the Pull-Up, put it in the plastic sealable bag, and close your overnight bag completely.

6. Get dressed and begin your day.

The following method works best if you don't have a place to change before you go to sleep:

1. Put a Pull-Up inside a pair of underpants or pajama bottoms, and place them at the bottom of your sleeping bag. Put a plastic bag in your sleeping bag as well.

2. When you're ready to go to sleep, get into your sleeping bag and wait 5 minutes or so for the bedtime chatter to quiet down.

3. Take off your underpants and push them to the side of your sleeping bag. Reach for your Pull-Up and slip it on with your boxers or pajama bottoms. If someone asks what you're doing, say you had an itch and were scratching your leg.

4. Consider having an adult wake you up around 6:00 or 7:00 am so you can take care of the Pull-Up before the other kids wake up.

5. After you wake up, remove the Pull-Up and put it in the plastic bag. Throw it away or push it to the bottom of your sleeping bag, whichever is easier to do. Put on your regular underpants, and go to the bathroom to pee.

6. If you were dry, you can stay in your sleeping bag for a while before getting up. If you were wet, roll up your sleeping bag right away and tie it closed.

7. Get dressed and begin your day.

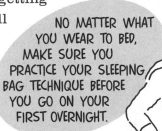

NO MATTER WHAT YOU WEAR TO BED, MAKE SURE YOU PRACTICE YOUR SLEEPING BAG TECHNIQUE BEFORE YOU GO ON YOUR FIRST OVERNIGHT.

Additional Tips for Going on Overnights

• Invite a friend to your house the first time you have a sleep-over. This will give you more confidence because you'll be in the comfort of your own home.

• The first time you have a sleepover at someone else's house, make sure it's one of your best friends. That way, if something goes wrong, you're in a better position to explain what happened without being teased.

• When children go to weeklong sleepaway camps, they usually stay in cabins. Sometimes they sleep in beds, and sometimes they sleep in sleeping bags on wooden platforms. In many cases, there won't be a bathroom in the cabin, so be prepared to use an outhouse if necessary.

• If you go to a weeklong camp, store the Pull-Ups in a pillow-case at the bottom of your overnight bag.

• Going to sleepaway camp for more than a week is tricky because you need more Pull-Ups and there's a greater chance someone will find out about your bedwetting. As a result, I usually recommend you postpone longer periods away from home until you've become dry at night.

• If you decide to go to sleepaway camp, one of your parents should talk to the camp director to find out if the camp has a policy for campers who are wet at night. Many camps make an extra effort to help kids with medical conditions.

FUN FACT

Unless you have a bladder infection, urine is *sterile*, which means it's free of germs. Your mouth, on the other hand, is a cesspool of germs!

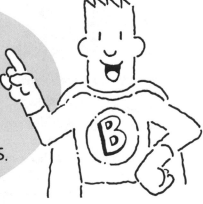

HERE'S ANOTHER IDEA FOR YOUR FIRST SLEEPOVER AWAY FROM HOME—INSTEAD OF GOING TO A FRIEND'S HOUSE, HAVE A PRACTICE SLEEPOVER WITH ONE OF YOUR RELATIVES.

Eric's Story

A few years ago, one of my 10-year-old patients went to a 4-week sleepover camp. Eric wet the bed most nights, and he was worried his bunkmates would find out. When his mom called the camp about Eric's concern, she was reassured that they dealt with this all the time.

On the first day of camp, Eric's counselor told the boys they had to take a shower every morning. He added that they would pick straws to decide the order in which they would use the shower.

Eric picked first, and he got the short straw. His counselor said, "Sorry, Eric, but you got the short straw, so I'll be waking you up before everyone else for the next 4 weeks." Eric put on a sulky face, but this had all been arranged ahead of time.

By waking up first, Eric had time to take care of his wet bed while the other kids were still asleep. His counselor helped by taking his wet sheets to the laundry while Eric showered. No one found out that he wet the bed.

COACH'S CORNER

My 9-year-old is going to camp in a few months, and his doctor recommended a medication called desmopressin. Is this a good idea?

Although desmopressin doesn't usually cure bedwetting, it definitely has a role to play in helping children stay dry at night. If your doctor recommends desmopressin, he or she will probably start with a low dose and work up depending on your child's response. However, keep in mind that it's only effective about 50% of the time. When I use desmopressin with my own patients, I like to see it work for 7 nights in a row before I'm confident it will do the job at camp. (See the Desmopressin section on pages 201–202 for ways to reduce the possibility of developing side effects from the medication.)

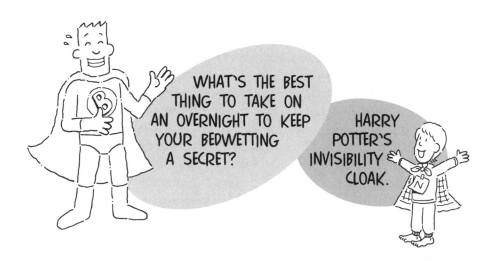

WHAT'S THE BEST THING TO TAKE ON AN OVERNIGHT TO KEEP YOUR BEDWETTING A SECRET?

HARRY POTTER'S INVISIBILITY CLOAK.

CHAPTER 23

What to Do if Someone Discovers Your Supplies

It's important to keep your bedwetting supplies in a safe place so no one finds them by accident and teases you or asks questions that might embarrass you. However, mistakes happen, so it's a good idea to be prepared ahead of time.

This chapter describes situations that may occur while you're doing the program and ways you can handle them. There are no "right" answers, so fill in the blank spaces if you can think of any others.

KID'S ALERT

I'm sure your parents have taught you how important it is to tell the truth. I agree with this completely. However, there are situations where I think it's OK to tell a white lie. Most of the time, people do this because they don't want to hurt someone's feelings. If your grandmother made a meal that tasted awful, would you tell her the truth or would you keep your thoughts to yourself? In my opinion, sparing your grandmother's feelings isn't the same as cheating on a test or lying about something you broke. I feel the same way about keeping your bedwetting a secret if that's what you've chosen to do. Please discuss my suggestions with your parents. If they disagree with my approach, I want you to follow their advice, not mine.

Someone Finds Your Calendar

- "I've been exercising lately, and I'm using the calendar to follow my progress." (You can add that *LW* stands for *long workout, SW* stands for *short workout,* and *D* stands for *day off.* The check marks are for those days when you worked out extra hard.)

- _____

- _____

Someone Finds a Stack of Pull-Ups in Your Bathroom

- "They're my sister's." (Get your sister's permission before using this excuse.)
- "My parents keep Pull-Ups on hand in case one of my cousins spends the night."

- _____

- _____

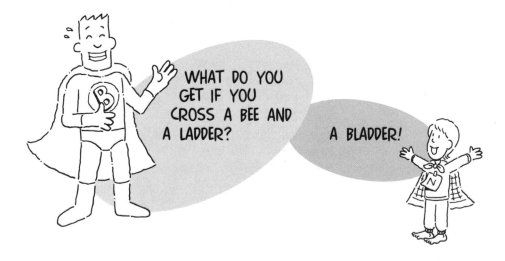

Someone Sees You in a Pull-Up

- "I have a bladder infection, and my doctor told me to wear a Pull-Up because urine can leak at night with this type of infection."

- _____

- _____

David's Story

When kids see me for their yearly checkups, I usually ask for a urine specimen to make sure their kidneys are healthy. Sometimes the nurses give them a urine cup before the examination, and sometimes I give it to them after. One day I handed the cup to a 6-year-old while I was still talking to his mom. As we sat there finishing up, David pulled down his pants and started peeing right before our eyes! Lucky for me, his aim was pretty good and he didn't overflow the cup.

Someone Notices You Were Wet at Night

- Same as previous answer.

- _____

- _____

Someone Sees an Underpad on Your Bed

- "I felt sick last night, and my parents put this on the bed in case I threw up."

- _____

- _____

Someone Finds Your Alarm

- "I've been having trouble waking up in the morning, and my parents bought a special buzzer to get me out of bed." (You can trigger the alarm to demonstrate how loud it is.)

- _____

- _____

Someone Finds Your _Waking Up Dry_ Book

- "One of my cousins had a sleepover last week and left the book at my house by mistake."
- "Oh, that's an old book. I had some trouble staying dry at night when I was little."

- _____

- _____

Someone Finds Your Medicine

"That's an allergy medicine I take at night."

_____

_____

CHAPTER 24

Lifting, Pull-Ups, & Other Measures

Lifting

One of the things parents do to help kids stay dry is take them to the bathroom a few hours after they go to sleep. This technique is called *lifting* because in many cases, children barely wake up and walk zombie-like to the bathroom. (In some cases, parents even carry their kids to the bathroom.) Lifting is not a treatment for bedwetting. Rather, it's a simple measure parents can use until you become dry on your own or you are ready to start a bedwetting program. Lifting isn't for everyone, however. Some children wet the bed 2 or 3 times a night, and I usually don't recommend waking kids multiple times to keep them dry. Also, parents need to consider your age. In general, I think lifting is OK for children between 4 and 8 years of age. There are a few situations in which it's OK for older kids to use lifting as a method to stay dry.

- Sleepovers
- Vacation
- If circumstances make it impossible for you to do the program
- As a temporary measure if you are setting off your alarm 2 or more times per night (see the Your Child Wets the Bed More Than Once per Night section on page 183.)
- If you don't become dry after doing the program

Taylor's Story

A few years ago, one of my patients came up with a great idea for taking her son to the bathroom at night. Instead of just waking him, she used a combination of waking up practice and the wake-up drill. As Taylor's mom got him out of bed, she said, "Wake up, Taylor. Your bladder is trying to wake you up. Taylor, your bladder is as big as an orange, and it's sending a signal to your brain telling you it's time to get up. You need to wake up if you want to have dry beds." Taylor's mom repeated this message as she tried to wake up her son. Some nights, Taylor's mom needed to shake his shoulders or sit him up to get him to wake up. Other nights, he woke up right away. When Taylor walked to the bathroom, his mom continued to talk to him: "Great job, Taylor. Your bladder sent a signal to your brain waking you up, and you're going to the bathroom to pee. You can do this every night if your bladder fills up with urine." After Taylor peed, his mom praised him for going to the bathroom and reminded him one more time that he would wake up if he needed to pee before morning.

Taylor's mom told me her efforts paid off. After a few months, he began waking up on his own if he needed to pee in the middle of the night.

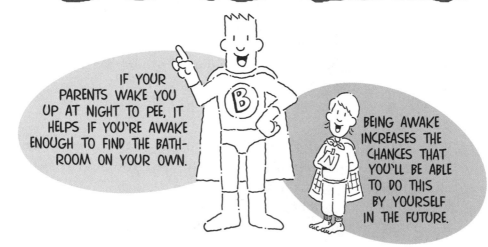

IF YOUR PARENTS WAKE YOU UP AT NIGHT TO PEE, IT HELPS IF YOU'RE AWAKE ENOUGH TO FIND THE BATHROOM ON YOUR OWN.

BEING AWAKE INCREASES THE CHANCES THAT YOU'LL BE ABLE TO DO THIS BY YOURSELF IN THE FUTURE.

FUN FACT The comedian Will Rogers once said that everything is funny as long as it happens to someone else. In that vein, I've heard lots of funny stories about lifting over the years. One of my patients was so sleepy when his parents woke him up one night that he peed in the garbage can instead of the toilet. Another patient fooled his parents one night when he looked like he was awake after they got him up to pee. He went to the bathroom, said good-night, and proceeded to get in bed with his sister. Fortunately, he was dry when he woke up the next morning. One of my female patients was taken to the bathroom at night, but no one noticed she forgot to pull down her underpants until it was too late!

Pull-Ups

One of the questions that comes up at bedwetting visits is what children should do about Pull-Ups. My approach to Pull-Ups is practical. If you're a 5- to 7-year-old who's not ready to do the program, it's OK to wear them. Once you turn 8, however, you should stop using Pull-Ups, even if you're not ready to do the program. Therefore, if you're older than 7 and you're not ready to work on the program, it's better to use underpads instead (see the Making It Easier to Deal With Wet Betting section on page 196). There are a few situations in which it's OK for older children to wear Pull-Ups, however.

- Overnights
- During an illness
- On vacation if you're sleeping at a hotel or someone else's house
- If something very important is coming up, such as a school play or special project, and you need to get a good night's sleep

Drinking After Dinner

Many people think that not drinking fluids after dinner helps children stay dry. Although this helps some children, it doesn't work for most. If you limit fluids, you may wet the bed with 4 ounces of urine instead of 6, but you're still wet. Like Pull-Ups, my approach to limiting fluids is practical. If a child tells me that limiting fluids helps her stay dry, I give it my OK. Otherwise, I generally don't recommend this approach. There are a few exceptions to this rule.

- If you go on a sleepover, it seems reasonable to do everything you can to be dry that night.
- If you take the medication desmopressin, it's important to limit how much you drink after dinner.

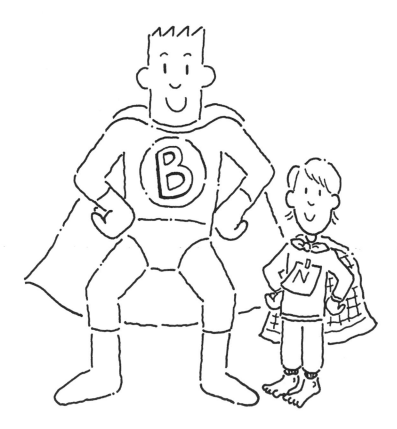

Word Search

```
W  A  K  I  N  G  U  P  P  R  A  C  T  I  C  E
S  P  W  M  Y  A  C  L  C  M  U  R  I  N  E  K
P  A  Q  O  X  B  H  D  K  B  O  I  D  G  F  Y
H  B  E  D  W  E  T  T  I  N  G  A  L  A  R  M
I  N  I  C  L  A  B  M  D  G  N  K  J  H  E  S
N  R  W  J  H  T  U  E  N  D  R  Y  B  E  D  L
C  P  Z  B  O  T  D  C  E  I  N  T  C  K  F  E
T  B  S  L  P  H  K  F  Y  E  L  X  O  Y  J  E
E  A  W  A  T  E  R  G  U  L  P  I  N  G  D  P
R  I  Y  D  N  B  W  V  M  P  F  J  T  C  Z  O
M  F  X  D  O  U  Q  G  R  E  W  A  R  D  S  V
U  J  V  E  K  Z  D  R  J  I  T  G  A  S  Q  E
S  A  U  R  T  Z  V  L  M  S  N  U  C  R  G  R
C  K  C  A  L  E  N  D  A  R  V  E  T  U  W  S
L  T  L  N  V  R  S  B  T  V  Q  R  W  I  Y  R
E  M  B  U  O  S  Y  O  U  C  A  N  D  O  I  T
```

BEAT THE BUZZER

BEDWETTING ALARM

BLADDER

CALENDAR

CONTRACT

DRY BED

KIDNEY

REWARDS

SLEEPOVERS

SPHINCTER MUSCLE

URINE

WAKING UP PRACTICE

WATER GULPING

YOU CAN DO IT

(The solution is on page 173.)

COACH'S CORNER

Do all doctors think lifting is an acceptable option for children?

Some bedwetting experts discourage lifting because they think it interferes with a child's ability to become dry by "training" her to pee at the same time every night. I disagree with this opinion for the following reason: because specialists only treat patients who continue to wet the bed, they never see cases in which lifting helped. My experience is different. I'm a pediatrician, so I see the whole range of children's wetting problems, including cases in which lifting was helpful.

Does my child have to be fully awake when we take him to the bathroom at night?

No one has studied this scientifically. On the one hand, it seems intuitive that becoming fully conscious would help a child learn to wake up on his own in the future. However, because many children are deep sleepers, it may be difficult to accomplish this. As always, I take a practical approach to the problem.

- If you can't fully awaken your child, help him out of bed, but encourage him to find the bathroom on his own. Stay close by to ensure he makes it to and from the bathroom safely.
- If your child resists your efforts, do not force him to get up. Try again in 15 minutes or follow the tips on page 178 to see if you can rouse him enough to cooperate. If this doesn't work, let him stay asleep.

When I take my 8-year-old to the bathroom at night, she doesn't always urinate.

When children go to the bathroom at night, sometimes they just sit there and nothing comes out. If this happens, encourage your child to sit on the toilet for a few minutes before you assume she can't go. It also helps to turn on the faucet because running water often stimulates children to pee.

Why do you recommend getting rid of Pull-Ups when a child turns 8?

I make this recommendation because I think Pull-Ups may prolong the time it takes to become dry at night. Although no one has researched this question, I've had some experience over the years that supports this opinion. For example, I've had a number of patients who became dry months after they stop using Pull-Ups. I've also had patients who did not become motivated to work on the program until they stopped wearing Pull-Ups.

Word Search Solution

```
W  A  K  I  N  G  U  P  P  R  A  C  T  I  C  E
S  P  W  M  Y  A  C  L  C  M  U  R  I  N  E  K
P  A  Q  O  X  B  H  D  K  B  O  I  D  G  F  Y
H  B  E  D  W  E  T  T  I  N  G  A  L  A  R  M
I  N  I  C  L  A  B  M  D  G  N  K  J  H  E  S
N  R  W  J  H  T  U  E  N  D  R  Y  B  E  D  L
C  P  Z  B  O  T  D  C  E  I  N  T  C  K  F  E
T  B  S  L  P  H  K  F  Y  E  L  X  O  Y  J  E
E  A  W  A  T  E  R  G  U  L  P  I  N  G  D  P
R  I  Y  D  N  B  W  V  M  P  F  J  T  C  Z  O
M  F  X  D  O  U  Q  G  R  E  W  A  R  D  S  V
U  J  V  E  K  Z  D  R  J  I  T  G  A  S  Q  E
S  A  U  R  T  Z  V  L  M  S  N  U  C  R  G  R
C  K  C  A  L  E  N  D  A  R  V  E  T  U  W  S
L  T  L  N  V  R  S  B  T  V  Q  R  W  I  Y  R
E  M  B  U  O  S  Y  O  U  C  A  N  D  O  I  T
```

PART 7

Extra Stuff for Parents

CHAPTER 25

Getting Past the Rough Spots

Becoming dry takes a lot of work, and the Waking Up Dry Program gets complicated at times. In addition, bedwetting alarms don't always work the way they're supposed to. One way to keep your child from quitting the program is to know what to do if you run into trouble along the way.

Your Child Doesn't Wake Up When the Alarm Goes Off

This is very common at the beginning of the program, which is why I recommend that parents sleep in the child's bedroom for the first 2 weeks they're using the alarm. Be sure to use the wake-up drill (see the How to Do the Wake-up Drill section on page 67) if you need help getting your child to wake up. Most kids begin waking up on their own a week or so into the program. If your child doesn't wake up at that point, consider using an alarm that vibrates in addition to buzzing.

Some parents can't sleep in their child's bedroom because it's too small, they have back problems, or other hurdles get in the way. In this case, get to your child's bedroom as quickly as possible after he wets the bed. Some bedwetting alarms have extra receivers that go in the parent's bedroom to help them wake up. Another option would be to use a baby monitor that will pick up the sound of the alarm in your child's room.

Your Child Is Sleepy or Grumpy When He Wakes Up

It's hard for anyone to be awakened from sleep, especially when an alarm is blaring in the background. Although most kids eventually learn to wake up, they may be groggy when the alarm goes off. There are a few things to consider in this situation.

Sometimes a child will utter things that don't make sense or say mean things to you. He also may turn over or push you away. This happens because he's disoriented or not fully awake. He may complain when you try to get him to the bathroom. If this happens, try to wake him using some of the techniques discussed in the How to Do the Wake-up Drill section on page 67. If you're unable to rouse him or he's still grumpy when he's awake, be patient but persistent. Concentrate on getting him to the bathroom to finish peeing in the toilet. Help him put on dry clothes, and reconnect the alarm. In the morning, compliment him on anything that went well the night before.

Sometimes a child wakes up and does what he's supposed to but is obviously in a dreamy state. My advice is this situation is practical. If your child is making progress with the program, continue as you are. If he's not making progress, rethink what you're doing. Go to his room as soon as the alarm buzzes, and try the following things to wake him:

• Talk to him with an animated tone, trying hard to get him to look you in the eye.
• Wet his face with a washcloth.
• Turn on the bedroom light.
• Turn on a radio, TV, or music player if one is available.

The Alarm Doesn't Go Off When Your Child Wets the Bed

This is a frustrating problem that can occur for a number of reasons.

- The sensor is in the wrong place. Although boys usually pee in the front of their underpants and girls at the bottom, this isn't always the case. If your child wakes up in a wet bed, but the alarm hasn't gone off, check to see if his underpants are wet where the sensor was located. If not, reposition the sensor on subsequent nights.

- The sensor shifts out of position or falls off because it doesn't have a good fit. This can happen for a few reasons: a child's underwear is too thick, or the sensor itself has loosened up over time. Girl's underwear is the usual cause for the first problem because it often has a double layer of fabric in the crotch area. If you can't find thin underwear, cut away the inner layer of fabric or use boy's underpants. This problem is most likely to occur with snap-on sensors and ones that attach to underpants with tape or panty liners. If the sensor has lost its grip, get a new one or purchase a different alarm.

- The sensor becomes detached because the child is an active sleeper. You can prevent this from happening by securing the sensor (or cord) to the child's bedclothes with a small clip or masking tape. This problem is less likely to occur with clip-on sensors.

- The battery is low, the sensor needs to be cleaned, or there is a problem with the alarm itself. Call the manufacturer or place of purchase if the alarm continues to malfunction after you replace the battery and clean the sensor.

Your Child Turns Off the Alarm and Goes Back to Sleep

Sometimes a child rouses just enough to unhook the sensor but then falls asleep instead of getting up and going to the bathroom. (If this happens, you may not hear the alarm and therefore won't know she wet the bed.) This is the reason why the best alarms have a 2-step process to turn them off: the child unhooks the sensor *and* pushes a button on the alarm box. The best way to determine if this is going on is to sleep in your child's room so you can monitor what happens after the alarm buzzes. If she disconnects the alarm in this fashion, wake her up every time it happens until she is getting up the way she's supposed to.

Your Child Has Trouble Turning Off the Alarm

Children sometimes have difficulty turning off bedwetting alarms, especially at the beginning of the program. There are a few reasons why this can occur.

- Most children are sleepy when they're woken up and may be all thumbs in the first week or so that they're using the alarm.
- Some children grab the cord instead of the sensor. If this happens, the cord will bend, making it harder to detach the sensor.
- Some alarms are harder to turn off than others. Clip-on sensors, which do an excellent job staying attached throughout the night, are also more difficult to unhook.

Encourage your child to practice turning off the alarm before she goes to sleep. If possible, she should do this while she's under the covers with the light turned off to simulate what happens at night. (Remember that night-lights make the program easier.) In most cases, her ability to turn off the alarm will improve with time. If she continues to have trouble, you can help her turn it off by guiding her through the process.

Children sometimes have difficulty getting the sensor back in place when they're sleepy. After a child wets the bed, she's supposed to get up and go to the bathroom to finish peeing. She then comes back to her bedroom, puts on new underpants, and reconnects the sensor. Some children have more difficulty attaching their alarm after a wetting episode than when they first went to bed. When this happens, it's OK to attach the sensor for your child.

Your Child Argues That He Didn't Wet the Bed

There are 2 situations when this can happen. First, a child can look at his underpants in the morning and argue that they're not wet. If this happens, encourage him to reread the Kid's Alert box on page 55. Second, a child can wake up after a wetting episode and do everything he's supposed to but not remember it happening when he wakes up the following day. If this happens, leave his wet bedding from the night before in his room. (Put it in a basket so it doesn't make the carpet smell.) That way, when he wakes up in the morning, he'll know he had a wet night without you having to say anything.

The Alarm Disturbs Family Members When It Goes Off

Most children don't want to draw attention to their bedwetting, and waking siblings doesn't help matters. There are some things you can do to remedy this situation. If your kids share a bedroom, it may help if you separate them until the program is over. The child doing the program should remain in his own bed, but you can let the other child use a bed, a sleeping bag, or a makeshift tent somewhere else. Try to make the adjustment sound like an adventure instead of an imposition.

If your children don't share a room, try to make the alarm's sound less noticeable. Play a radio or sound machine in the second child's room, or lower the sound of the alarm if possible. You can do this by putting a piece of tape over the speaker or turning down the volume if that option is available. A vibrating alarm (with the sound turned off) may also work as long as it consistently wakes your child when it goes off.

The Alarm Disturbs Your Neighbors When It Goes Off

This is similar to the situation just described, but the solution is trickier because it involves neighbors instead of family members. You may be able to solve the problem by having your child move to another bedroom. If another room isn't available, consider putting your child's mattress somewhere else in the apartment. If neither of these options is feasible, you can reduce the alarm's sound by putting a piece of tape over the speaker or turning down the volume if that option is available. Obviously, the sound needs to be loud enough to wake the child. As previously noted, a vibrating alarm may solve the problem. It may help if you tell your neighbors why an alarm is going off in your apartment at night. (A bottle of wine or other gift may also help smooth things over.)

Your Child Isn't Cooperating With the Program

If your child isn't cooperating with the program, the first thing you should do is take a deep breath and try not to get upset. Then pay attention to what he's doing for a few days. If he's forgetting (or refusing) to do some of his work, talk to him in a relaxed manner so you can find out why he's acting the way he is. Here are some reasons why a child may stop cooperating with the program.

- He's distracted by schoolwork, sports, or other interests. Address his concerns, and point out how they are interfering with the program. Brainstorm solutions to the problems, and see if there's anything you can do to help.
- The program is too complicated. Simplify things by reducing the frequency of an exercise or eliminating it altogether.
- He's forgetful. (This is especially true for kids with attention-deficit/hyperactivity disorder.) Try to come up with some ways to remind him what to do without his feeling like you're nagging. Some kids prefer to be reminded verbally. Others respond better if you hand them a note or put a reminder in their room. (You can use the Waking Up Dry checklist on page 210.)
- He may be frustrated because the program isn't working fast enough. Look at his calendar to see if he's making progress such as smaller wet spots, waking up quicker when the alarm goes off, and peeing later in the night. Reread Chapter 15 together; it's a pep talk from me to your child.
- He's uncooperative when the alarm goes off. Children sometimes get frustrated when the alarm wakes them up night after night. Make sure you're doing everything you can to simplify what happens when the alarm goes off. (See Chapter 26 for tips on making it easier to deal with wet beds in the middle of the night.)
- He may be having false alarms, or the alarm may not be working properly. Do what you can to fix these problems.

Your Child Wets the Bed More Than Once per Night

If the alarm goes off more than once a night, it can create a few problems. First, you and your child will lose a lot of sleep. Second, your child is more likely to become discouraged about the program. How you approach this depends on the number of times the alarm goes off. If it goes off twice a night and your child can handle the situation, continue with the program as before. If it goes off more than twice a night or your child is getting frustrated, consider the following options. (Once your child begins responding to the program, you can stop these measures and go back to using the alarm the regular way.)

- Have your child urinate twice before he goes to sleep. Ask him to go 30 minutes before bed and again when he does his waking up practice.
- Take your child to the bathroom before you go to sleep. Emptying his bladder at 10:00 or 11:00 pm may reduce the number of times the alarm goes off.
- Stop using the alarm after it goes off for the second time. Although your child could wet the bed a third time, this may be a better option than becoming exhausted at the beginning of the program.
- Talk with your doctor about adding a medicine to the program. Depending on the size of your child's bladder, there are different medications that can reduce the number of wettings per night (see Chapter 27).

False Alarms

This doesn't happen often, but it's very frustrating when it does. Here are the reasons why false alarms occur.

- If your child uses an alarm that snaps or clips to his underpants, the metal parts of the sensor may touch each other if there are tiny holes in the fabric. If this happens, the alarm will go off even though the underpants are dry. To fix this problem, examine your child's underpants, and throw away the "bad" ones or put them in a special drawer so they're not used with the alarm.

- There are 2 conditions that may result in a small amount of urine leaking into a child's underpants at night. The first condition occurs in girls. Sometimes when girls pee, a small amount of urine goes into the vagina instead of the toilet. If this happens, the urine can leak out when they're in bed and set off the alarm. Girls can fix this problem by separating their legs when they pee or by sitting on the toilet backward. (This keeps their legs apart, which prevents urine from getting into the vagina.) The second condition occurs in boys who are not circumcised. Most uncircumcised boys do not pull their foreskin back when they pee. If urine gets trapped in the foreskin, it can leak out when they're in bed and set off the alarm. Boys can fix this problem by pulling their foreskin back when they pee and shaking off any drops of urine that remain on the end of the penis.

- If a child sweats a lot, perspiration can wet the sensor and set off the alarm. You can fix this problem by making the room a little cooler or by having your child sleep with fewer blankets. If this doesn't work, your child can wear a second pair of underpants inside the pair with the sensor. If this doesn't solve the problem, try a different alarm.

- False alarms can also occur if the battery is low; the sensor needs to be cleaned, or the alarm isn't working properly.

Getting Sick During the Program

If your child gets a minor illness, such as a cold, you should continue with the program. If she develops something worse, it's OK to stop until she is well. You can use Pull-Ups during the illness if it makes her feel better or your morning routine easier.

Feeling Discouraged About the Program

Sometimes it feels like it's taking forever to start having dry nights. If your child thinks this is happening, check her calendar to see if she's making progress. If she isn't making progress, follow the suggestions in the next section. If she is making progress, remind your child what I said about learning a new skill. It takes time, patience, and practice for things to pay off. Reread Chapter 15 together; it's a pep talk from me to your child.

Your Child Isn't Making Progress With the Program

You can measure progress with the program in 5 different ways. Your child wakes up on his own when the alarm goes off.
• He has smaller wet spots.
• He has fewer wet episodes per night. (Most kids wet the bed once per night. If your child wets the bed more frequently, you can use this to measure his progress.)
• He has more dry nights.
• He wets later in the night.

   The following options are for 2 groups of kids: those who have made no progress 4 weeks into the program and those who made some progress initially but continue to have mostly wet nights 6 to 8 weeks into the program.
• If your child didn't do water gulping when he began the program, do it now.
• When your child does waking up practice (see page 84), have him go to the bathroom twice instead of once. The first time he sits on the toilet, he should just pretend to pee.
• Talk to your doctor about adding a medicine to the program. There are a few medications that may help by reducing the number of wettings per night.

• If none of these options work, continue with the program for another 8 weeks. If your child is still not making progress, talk to your doctor or take a break and try the program again in 6 to 12 months.

Parents Become Frustrated With the Program or Each Other

Although children do the most work to become dry at night, the program is hard on parents as well. The following situations (and solutions) are the ones I deal with most often in my office.

The alarm is too much of an intrusion given the parents' current work situation.

1. Alternate responsibility for which parent gets up at night when the alarm goes off.

2. Postpone the program until the summer when most parents can slow down a bit at work.

3. Encourage your child to do the Modified Waking Up Dry Program discussed on page 79.

4. Have your child use an alarm clock to get him up at night. He can set the clock to go off once or twice a night depending on his wetting pattern (see the Coach's Corner box on page 74 for a comment on the Wake Assure alarm clock.)

5. If your child responds to the medication desmopressin, you can use this for sleepovers and other circumstances where he needs to be dry.

The parents agreed work together, but one of them sleeps through the alarm.

- Use a bedwetting alarm that has a remote receiver, or use a baby monitor in your bedroom, turned up high, right next to the less responsive parent. The other parent can use earplugs to suppress the sound of the alarm.
- The less responsive parent can sleep in the child's bedroom when it's his or her turn to supervise. This will make it easier to hear the alarm.
- One parent assumes nighttime alarm duty, while the other takes on other household responsibilities.

Dealing With Relapses

Learning to become dry is complicated. As a result, some children will wet the bed after they have reached their goal of 14 dry nights in a row. Having an occasional bedwetting is nothing to worry about, and a calm and reassuring attitude on your part will help prevent your child from losing her confidence and sense of pride over her recent accomplishments. It also helps to remind your child of all the progress she's made during the program. What you do about a relapse depends on when it happens and how often your child wets the bed. (If your child needs to restart the program, let her vent her frustrations for a while. Then try to bolster her motivation to work on the program.)

- If your child has any wet nights during the "cooling down" period, restart the program as described in the Finishing the Program section on page 140.
- If your child starts wetting the bed after the program is over, what you do depends on how often she wets the bed.
- If she wets the bed less than once a week, keep track of her wet and dry nights with the Waking Up Dry calendar.

- If she wets the bed once a week, have your child use the calendar and restart her waking up practice. If she stops having accidents, continue with this plan for 3 more weeks. If the wetting continues, follow the recommendations in the next step.
- If she wets the bed more than once a week, restart the program. Once she's been dry for 14 nights in a row, add a technique called **overlearning.**

Overlearning is a procedure that strengthens what your child learns with the bedwetting alarm. The technique involves drinking a 6- to 8-ounce glass of water right before going to sleep at night. In most cases, drinking this amount of water before bed will cause your child to start wetting again. This is normal, so don't let it discourage your child. She should continue to drink the water every night and use the alarm until she's been dry again for 14 nights in a row. Stop drinking the extra water and begin the "cooling down" period the same way she did with the regular program. When she finishes the program this time, her chances of having another relapse are very low (see the Coach's Corner box on page 193).

A GOOD WAY TO THINK ABOUT OVERLEARNING IS TO IMAGINE FAMOUS ATHLETES WHO CONTINUE TO PRACTICE AFTER THE REST OF THEIR TEAMMATES HAVE GONE HOME. THAT'S WHAT OVERLEARNING IS— REALLY HARD WORK TO HELP YOU STAY DRY AT NIGHT!

COACH'S CORNER

Should my daughter lose her weekly reward if she doesn't cooperate with the program?

The reason I recommend weekly rewards is to motivate children to stick with the program, especially if they're not having success right away. If a child stops cooperating with the program, the first thing to do is to find out why this is happening (see Your Child Isn't Cooperating With the Program on page 182). If you don't turn up anything after this inquiry, review which rewards she's earned so far and which ones are still to come. If this doesn't motivate her, gently remind her what she agreed to do when she signed the Waking Up Dry contract. If this doesn't work, you should go ahead and withhold one of her weekly rewards. Remember to do this without expressing any anger or frustration, which would only sour her attitude toward the program. In a day or so, ask her if she's ready to continue with the program.

My son has always been wet at night. When we began the program, he had 5 dry nights in the first week. Now he's been wet 4 nights in a row, and he's very disappointed.

This is similar to the **honeymoon period** described in the Coach's Corner box on page 50. I suspect your son had his initial run of dry nights because his excitement about the program altered his sleep habits. Now that the program is in full swing, he's gone back to his regular sleep pattern, and the reality of the hard work he'll need to do is staring him in the face. It's important to let him know this happens to lots of kids. Tell him that having 5 dry nights proves he can beat the problem but that it will take time for his brain and bladder to learn how to talk to each other every night.

My daughter has been using the Malem Ultimate for 3 weeks. If she wakes up at night to pee (when the alarm hasn't gone off), it's hard for her to reattach the sensor by herself.

Children sometimes have difficulty getting the sensor back in place when they're sleepy. If kids get up at night to pee, they can avoid this problem by not unhooking the sensor before they go. There are 2 ways to accomplish this. The first involves pulling the bottom of her underpants to one side before urinating. After your daughter pees, she can wipe herself with one hand while she continues to hold her underpants out of the way. It's important she wipes herself well so the alarm doesn't go off because urine leaks out of the vaginal area after she gets in bed. The second option involves carefully pulling down the underpants with the sensor still attached. As long as there is a little slack in the cord or the child leans forward, the sensor shouldn't come off during this maneuver.

My 11-year-old has been using the alarm for 6 weeks and is now having dry nights half the time. Although he's cooperating with the program, he says he hates his alarm.

This is a common reaction in older kids. When your son says he hates his alarm, what he probably means is he hates that he wets the bed and resents having to do all the extra work to become dry at night. The alarm is a symbol for his problem and therefore the focus of his frustration. Avoid the pitfall of saying something like, "How can you hate your alarm when it's helping you become dry?" Instead, say something that reads between the lines: "It must be frustrating to have to work so hard to be dry at night." This may open a channel for further discussion, or it may just let him know you understand what he's going through.

continued on next page

My son started the program 6 weeks ago. He's doing great so far, but we have an unexpected beach vacation coming up, and we're worried about what will happen while we're away.

It's not uncommon that vacations have a way of creeping into the program. The big question, of course, is whether you continue with the alarm while you're away. In general, it's a good idea to stick with the program if you can. One option is to have him wear Pull-Ups over his briefs. That way, he can still use the alarm, but you'll have no clean up to do. Keep in mind that children are usually tired during vacations, and it may be difficult to keep up with the rest of the program. Therefore, it's reasonable to limit him to the alarm and the calendar to monitor his progress.

My son has been doing a great job with the program, but he wet the bed last night after 12 dry nights in a row. He's pretty disappointed, and we're not sure how to handle it.

This is hard on kids, but it happens sometimes. The key thing is acknowledging your child's feelings while trying to keep him motivated to stick with the program. Rather than repeat what I said in Chapter 15, I thought it would help if I wrote a mock dialogue that addresses your question. (I know that real life isn't this simple, but I hope it gives you an idea of how to approach the problem.)

Parent: What's the matter?

Child: I wet the bed last night.

Parent: You look disappointed.

Child: Wouldn't you be?

Parent: Sure I would. I'd feel lousy.

Child: When is this going to stop?

Parent: I'm not sure when you'll be dry for good, but I know you've been doing a great job with the program.

Child: Then how come I'm still wet?

Parent: Because it takes time to learn to be dry. Don't forget, you've been wet at night your whole life. Your body can't learn what it's supposed to do right away.

Child: I'm just so sick of it! When I wake up in a wet bed, I just think, "Oh no, not again. How can this be happening again?"

Parent: Well, for one thing, it's not because you're not trying. Sometimes kids just don't wake up when they need to pee. Remember when I was learning to ski last year? I must have fallen down a hundred times before I got it right.

Child: I remember. Your nose was so red it looked like a strawberry. Come to think of it, I am waking up more on my own the past few weeks.

Parent: Exactly. You wake up all the time when the alarm goes off and lots of times when it doesn't. I'm really proud of how well you're doing.

Child: But I was so close to earning my special reward! Now it feels like it'll be months before I get it.

Parent: It may seem like forever, but it won't be. Hey, I've got an idea. Let's review all of the weekly rewards you've earned since you started the program.

Child: OK. I'll get my calendar.

My 10-year-old has used the alarm twice in the past year, but she relapses every time we finish the program. We even tried overlearning, but nothing has kept her consistently dry.

This doesn't happen very often, but I occasionally see children who relapse after they do the overlearning procedure.

continued on next page

I mentioned earlier that most kids who become dry with the alarm eventually learn to sleep until morning and don't need to wake up at night to pee. Children who relapse over and over usually have small bladders and are not able to hold their urine until morning. When these kids become dry, it's because the alarm teaches them to wake up when their bladders get full. Then, for some reason, they lose this skill weeks or months after the program is over. The only way these kids will stay dry is to consistently wake up when their bladders fill up at night. The first thing I'd recommend is for you to sit down with your daughter and encourage her to voice her frustrations about what's been happening. Once you've sympathized with her situation, there are a few options to consider.

- The next time you do the program, use the alarm until she's been dry for 30 nights in a row.
- *Hypnotherapy,* or medical hypnosis, is a technique that uses visualization, imagery, and posthypnotic suggestions to help people with many conditions (eg, to stop smoking, to lose weight, to manage chronic pain). Hypnotherapy can also be used to treat bedwetting. It works by giving your child posthypnotic "suggestions" to awaken if her bladder fills up with urine during the night. If this sounds interesting to you, ask your doctor for the name of an appropriate therapist in your area.
- Ask your doctor about using a medication like desmopressin to stay dry.
- Have your daughter take a 6- to 12-month break from the program. During this time, institute a scheduled lifting program, with 1 or 2 awakenings per night to help her stay dry.

CHAPTER 26

Tips for Dealing With Wet Beds

For most children, the best thing about becoming dry is no longer having to wake up in a wet bed. The second best thing is being able to go on sleepovers without worrying about what will happen during the night. Because it takes time for the program to work, you and your child will need to deal with wet beds for a while longer. The purpose of this chapter is to teach you some practical tips that will make your morning routine easier. Although you're probably doing some of these things already, there are 4 areas I want to review.

• Protecting your child's mattress and pillow
• Making it easier to deal with wet bedding
• Getting rid of unpleasant urine smells in your child's room
• Supplies to have on hand

Protecting Your Child's Mattress and Pillow

When a child wets the bed, urine can leak through the sheets and into the mattress. Over time, the mattress will start to smell like urine. To prevent this from happening, you should protect your child's mattress with a waterproof cover. Mattress covers protect the top and sides of the mattress or encase it completely. Pillows are less likely to get wet at night, but washable pillows and waterproof pillow covers are also available. You can buy mattress and pillow covers at department stores or from online medical supply companies that sell bedwetting products. Cheap mattress covers may crack or leak, so try to find one that's well made.

Making It Easier to Deal With Wet Bedding

One way to make your mornings easier is to put a protective pad on your child's sheets. These products, called *underpads*, come in 2 basic styles—reusable and disposable. Reusable underpads have cloth on one side and a waterproof backing on the other. Disposable underpads have absorbent material on one side and a thin plastic layer on the other. The reusable type costs more to begin with, but they're less expensive over time because you wash them over and over. Disposable underpads are more expensive over time because they're made to be used once and thrown away. Although they cost more, disposable underpads are easier to use because you don't have to wash them.

Disposable underpads come in different sizes and thicknesses. There are 3 basic sizes you will find—23 x 36 inches, 30 x 30 inches, and 30 x 36 inches. The advantage of the bigger sizes is they cover a larger area, so your child is less likely to miss the pad if he tosses and turns while he sleeps. Which thickness to buy is a matter of personal preference. Thinner pads (light absorbency) cost less and will do the job for most children. If your child produces a lot of urine at night, you can always move up to a thicker pad (moderate or heavy absorbency).

Some disposable underpads come with an adhesive strip on the back to keep them in place at night. Another brand, called Tuckables, have extra-long plastic wings that are tucked under the mattress. (Tuckables are 70 inches wide, but the extra length is in the wings, not the pad.) In my experience, most children are too active at night for any underpad to stay put. Fortunately, there is a solution to this problem.

Keeping Disposable Underpads In Place

The easiest way to keep underpads from moving around is to layer them between fitted sheets. Make your child's bed as follows:

1. Put on the bottom fitted sheet.

2. Place an underpad on top of the sheet in the middle of the bed.

3. Put a second fitted sheet on top of the bottom sheet, making sure the underpad stays in place.

4. Place an underpad on top of the second fitted sheet.

5. Put a third fitted sheet on top of the second sheet, making sure the underpad stays in place.

This layering technique serves 2 purposes. First, it will keep the underpads from moving around. Second, if your child wets the bed, you can remove the top sheet and the wet underpad that's underneath it. You won't have to remake the bed because another fitted sheet and underpad are already in place.

If you don't have enough sheets to use the layering technique, you can keep underpads in place by taping them to a fitted sheet with 4 pieces of 2-inch masking tape. In this case, your child will sleep on top of the underpad. If your child has a dry night, you don't need to change her underpad in the morning. In fact, if she has a run of dry nights, most underpads will last for about a week. After that, the absorbent layer gets tattered and needs to be changed. (If your child doesn't use the layering technique, remind her to make the bed every morning so no one sees the underpad.)

You can buy underpads at most pharmacies and from online medical supply companies. Online shopping gives you a bigger selection and is usually less expensive because you can buy products in bulk. Pharmacies have the advantage of being close to home.

Getting Rid of Unpleasant Urine Smells in Your Child's Room

Bedrooms can pick up a urine smell even if you take care of wet beds right away. Therefore, it's a good idea to have a backup plan in case you need it. The easiest way to handle any odor is with room freshener. There are many types available, but they all work by putting a pleasant smell in the air. You can buy room freshener at pharmacies and grocery stores.

Another way to handle urine smells is to use a product that eliminates odors instead of masking them. These products come as sprays and solid odor absorbers and are available from online medical supply companies. A great option for getting urine smells out of carpets is a product called Nature's Miracle, which is sold in pet stores. Although it's made for eliminating cat and dog smells, it works for people odors as well.

Supplies to Have on Hand

The program will run more smoothly if you always have plenty of basic supplies on hand. These include disposable products as well as clean undergarments and sheets. Here is a list of things you'll need.
• Mattress and pillow covers (Most children don't need pillow covers.)
• Sheets, blankets, and comforters
• Underpants

- Undershirts or pajama tops
- Pillowcases
- Underpads
- Two-inch masking tape
- Pull-Ups (for younger children and special circumstances)
- Odor eliminators
- Wipes (These come in handy when a bottom needs to be cleaned but your child doesn't have time for a morning bath or shower.)

Bedwetting Supply Companies

The easiest way to buy disposable underpads and other supplies is to search for the appropriate term on the Internet. There are 2 companies online that sell a wide variety of bedwetting products: PottyMD and the Bedwetting Store.

PottyMD
6804 Baum Drive
Knoxville, TN 37919
877/768-8963
www.pottymd.com

Bedwetting Store
11840 W Market Place Ste H
Fulton, MD 20759
800/214-9605
www.bedwettingstore.com

FUN FACT

Have you ever seen a kidney bean? Most kids don't like beans and go to great lengths to avoid eating them. But how about chili? Along with beef and tomato sauce, kidney beans are one of the main ingredients in chili. Kidney beans are about a half an inch long and pushed in on one side just like a kidney (see the How Do the Kidneys Make Urine? section on page 13). So which was named first, kidneys or kidney beans? The answer is the kidney. Believe it or not, the kidney was first named about 700 years ago. The kidney bean got its name 250 years later because someone noticed it looked a lot like the kidney.

CHAPTER 27

Medication

There are a few medications that doctors use to treat bedwetting. Although the goal of this book is to address the problem
without drugs, medication sometimes plays a role in helping
children become dry at night. Therefore, I thought it would be
useful to provide some information about these treatments.

Desmopressin (Brand Name: DDAVP)

The pituitary gland releases a hormone at night called *vasopressin* (VASE-oh-PRESS-in) that reduces the amount of urine
the kidneys make. (It does this by reabsorbing water from the
urine back into the bloodstream.) Although the research in
this area is inconclusive, it appears that some children wet
the bed because they don't make enough of this chemical.
Desmopressin is a manufactured form of vasopressin that
corrects this imbalance. The drug helps 50% of children who
take it, though research suggests it's less effective in patients
who have small bladders. The effects of desmopressin are not
long lasting, and children usually relapse when the drug is
stopped. For this reason, doctors generally recommend it for
short-term use (eg, sleepovers, vacations, special occasions).
Desmopressin is also useful if children are not making progress
with the program (see Chapter 25). Finally, a 6-month course
of desmopressin is worth considering in children who don't
become dry with the bedwetting alarm but need some treatment
that will get their wetting under control. (Recent research suggests it's safe to use desmopressin for longer periods of time.)

Although desmopressin does not cure bedwetting, it's a safe medication when used as directed. That said, the following concerns should be noted:

- There is a small risk that desmopressin will lower the sodium (salt) in a child's blood, which, in rare cases, can cause a seizure. This risk is greatly reduced if you limit a child's fluid intake on nights when he takes the medication. (Early symptoms of low sodium include headache, irritability, nausea, and vomiting.)
- Your child can have a 6- to 8-ounce glass of liquid after dinner, but he should avoid drinking more than a few sips within 2 hours of bedtime.
- If your child has an illness that requires extra fluid, stop the desmopressin until he is well. Also, withhold the medication if your child is doing the overlearning technique or has an unusually large fluid intake during the day.
- If your child is impulsive, make sure he doesn't drink water without your knowledge.
- Desmopressin is not a treatment for daytime wetting and therefore should never be used to correct this condition.

Oxybutynin (Brand Name: Ditropan)

Oxybutynin is usually prescribed for patients with an overactive bladder. People with an overactive bladder get uncontrolled bladder contractions that cause frequent urination and an urgent need to empty their bladders without much warning. Children with this problem have a small bladder capacity and often wet their beds more than once a night (many children with an overactive bladder have daytime wetting as well). Oxybutynin is not an effective treatment for bedwetting by itself. However, when used in conjunction with the bedwetting alarm, it may relax the bladder enough to make the alarm more successful. Therefore, if your child has these symptoms, talk with your doctor before starting the program or, alternatively, if you're not making progress by the time you are 4 weeks into treatment.

Although oxybutynin is generally a safe medication, like any drug, there are possible adverse effects. The most common side effects are dry mouth and facial flushing. Less frequent side effects include abdominal pain, constipation, and irritability.

Imipramine (Brand Name: Tofranil)

Imipramine was originally developed as a treatment for depression, but doctors discovered that people who took the drug sometimes had trouble emptying their bladders. This gave someone the idea that it might work with bedwetting. Recent studies suggest that imipramine may also affect a child's sleep, making her more aware of her bladder signals at night. Although the drug helps 40% of children who wet the bed, most relapse once the medication is stopped. More importantly, the difference between therapeutic and dangerous levels in the blood is small. As a result, many doctors (me included) are concerned that imipramine isn't safe enough to use in a benign condition such as bedwetting. Doctors that prescribe imipramine do not generally consider it a first-line treatment and only use it if other approaches fail.

Patient's Story

Many years ago, I read about an 8-year-old who died after taking an overdose of imipramine. No one knew exactly what happened, but it was assumed he took the overdose in an attempt to cure his bedwetting once and for all.

If anyone prescribes imipramine or any other medication for your child, be sure to tell him it is very dangerous to take more than what the doctor ordered. You should also lock it up so it doesn't get into the hands of small children.

CHAPTER 28

Bedwetting Treatment According to Age

Table 28-1 summarizes which aspects of the program are appropriate for children at different ages. The word *yes* does not mean you're obligated to do that part of the program, as there are other factors that will determine how you proceed. Yes simply means that a particular task is suitable for someone that age. The word *maybe* implies that it may or may not be a good idea to do that part of the program, so you need to individualize for your particular child. For example, few 6-year-olds are good candidates for the bedwetting alarm. Nevertheless, I have used

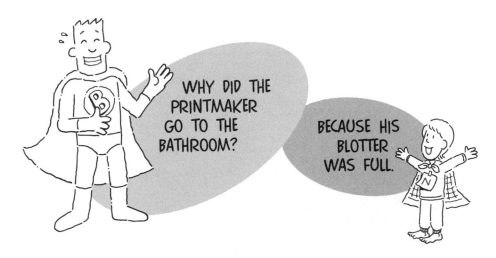

WHY DID THE PRINTMAKER GO TO THE BATHROOM?

BECAUSE HIS BLOTTER WAS FULL.

the alarm with kids this age, so there is no reason to prevent a highly motivated child from using it.

Table 28-1.
Bedwetting Treatment According to Age

Child's Age (years)	6–7	8–9	10+
Education[a]	Yes	Yes	Yes
Practical tip[b]	Yes	Yes	Yes
Lifting[c]	Yes	Maybe	Maybe
Pull-Ups at night[c]	Yes	Maybe	Maybe
Calendar & praise[d]	Yes	Yes	Yes
Bladder exercises			
Water gulping	Yes	Yes	Yes
Bladder attention	Yes	Yes	Yes
Waking up practice	Yes	Yes	Yes
Bedwetting alarm[e]	Maybe	Yes	Yes
Medication			
Desmopressin	Maybe	Yes	Yes
Oxybutynin	Maybe	Yes	Yes
Imipramine[f]	No	No	Maybe

[a] Education means reading the first part of the book with your child and teaching her how her body works. Kids are usually interested in their bodies and love doing the balloon experiment in Chapter 2.

[b] This refers to some of the basic things you do to make it easier to deal with wet beds, such as sheet protectors and extra bedding (see Chapter 26).

[c] I don't recommend lifting or Pull-Ups for older children except in special circumstances (see Chapter 24).

[d] Younger children may need help with their calendar, and they often prefer stickers instead of writing *D* after they've had a dry night.

[e] Most children 7 years and older can understand the purpose for the alarm and therefore can accept its negative consequences (eg, getting woken up at night). A few 6-year-olds may be suitable candidates if they are highly motivated.

[f] I don't use imipramine with children, but some doctors find it helpful for older patients who have not responded to other measures.

Appendixes

Waking Up Dry Checklist

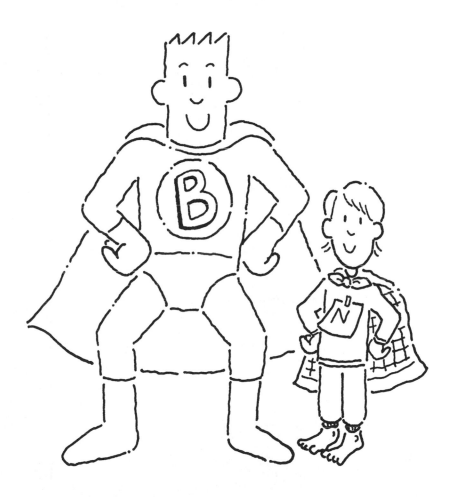

Day of the Week	Sunday	Monday	Tuesday	Wednesday	Thursday	Friday	Saturday
Month & Date	___	___	___	___	___	___	___
Water gulping	☐	☐	☐	☐	☐	☐	☐
	☐	☐	☐	☐	☐	☐	☐
Bladder attention	☐	☐	☐	☐	☐	☐	☐
	☐	☐	☐	☐	☐	☐	☐
	☐	☐	☐	☐	☐	☐	☐
	☐	☐	☐	☐	☐	☐	☐
Waking up practice	☐	☐	☐	☐	☐	☐	☐

Every time you do one of your exercises, mark the appropriate box. If you're unable to fill out the checklist during the day, record what you do before you go to sleep at night. Permission to reproduce for noncommercial purposes granted with acknowledgment. For all other purposes, please contact the American Academy of Pediatrics to request permission.

Health Screening Questionnaire

1. Has your child ever had a bladder or kidney infection? ☐ Yes ☐ No

2. Does your child complain of pain or burning when urinating? ☐ Yes ☐ No

3. Does your child urinate more than 9 times a day? ☐ Yes ☐ No

4. Does your child hold back urine for extended periods of time (ie, more than 8 hours)? ☐ Yes ☐ No

5. Does your child have daytime wetting? (This includes having damp underpants throughout the day.) ☐ Yes ☐ No

6. Has your child recently begun wetting the bed after 6 months or more of being dry at night? ☐ Yes ☐ No

7. Does your child have trouble with his urinary stream? (This includes dribbling, having a weak stream, or having to push hard to start urination.) ☐ Yes ☐ No

8. Does your child have damp underpants after going to the bathroom? ☐ Yes ☐ No

9. Does your child wake up more than once
a night to drink water? ☐ Yes ☐ No

10. Does your child have a problem with
abdominal pain or chronic diarrhea? ☐ Yes ☐ No

11. Does your child hold in bowel movements? ☐ Yes ☐ No

12. Does your child ever soil underpants
with stool? ☐ Yes ☐ No

13. Has your child experienced a recent
history of mood swings or other
emotional problems? ☐ Yes ☐ No

14. Does your child snore heavily at night in
such a way that your child sometimes
stops breathing or struggles to breathe? ☐ Yes ☐ No

15. Does your child have insomnia,
sleepwalking, or night terrors? ☐ Yes ☐ No

If you answered yes to any of these questions, do not begin the
program without seeing your doctor.

Bedwetting Questionnaire

I included this questionnaire in case you decide to do the Waking Up Dry Program with your doctor. These questions explore your wetting history and those parts of your life that may affect the program.

There are a lot of questions, so it's OK to ask your coaches for help. They can fill out the form for you, and they can answer any questions you're not sure of. (The questionnaire your coaches filled out to check for medical causes of bedwetting is in Appendix B. Bring both questionnaires to your visit.)

1. Date

   _____

2. Your name

   _____

3. Your age

   _____

4. What grade are you in?

   _____

5. What is your teacher's name? (If you have more than one teacher, write the name of the one you like best.)

   _____

6. What are your favorite subjects at school? (You can't pick recess!)

_____

7. Are you having any difficulties at school
   that might interfere with your staying
   focused on the program? ☐ Yes ☐ No

8. If you answered yes, what are they?

_____

_____

_____

9. What are your favorite hobbies?

_____

10. What are your favorite sports?

_____

11. Name one of your heroes or someone you look up to.

_____

12. Has anyone in your family had to work
    hard to overcome a problem in his or
    her life? ☐ Yes ☐ No

13. If you answered yes, who was it and what did he or
    she overcome?

_____

_____

14. Do you live in a house or an apartment?

_____

15. If you live in an apartment, do your next-door
    neighbors have children? ☐ Yes ☐ No

16. Is it possible your neighbors would hear
    the bedwetting alarm if it goes off at night? ☐ Yes ☐ No

17. Do you have your own bedroom? ☐ Yes ☐ No

18. If you have to share a bedroom, whom do you share it with?

    _____

19. Do you sleep in a bunk bed? ☐ Yes ☐ No

20. Is your bedroom located near your
    parent's bedroom? ☐ Yes ☐ No

21. If you answered no, where is your bedroom located?

    _____

22. Is your bedroom located near a bathroom? ☐ Yes ☐ No

23. If you answered no, where is the bathroom located?

    _____

24. Do you have carpeting in your bedroom? ☐ Yes ☐ No

25. Do you have carpeting in the hallway that
    leads to the bathroom? ☐ Yes ☐ No

26. Do you use a night-light or other light
    when you go to sleep at night? ☐ Yes ☐ No

27. Has anyone in your family ever wet the
    bed? (This includes parents, grandparents,
    siblings, and aunts and uncles.) ☐ Yes ☐ No

28. If you answered yes, who was it?

    _____

29. Does anyone outside of the family know
    you wet the bed? ☐ Yes ☐ No

30. If you answered yes, who is it and what is his or her
    relationship to you?

    _____

31. Is there anything your friends or family have done about your bedwetting that has bothered you (eg, teasing you, threatening to tell people you wet the bed)? ☐ Yes ☐ No

32. If you answered yes, what happened?

_____

_____

_____

33. Have your parents restricted you in any way because of your bedwetting (eg, not buying you a new mattress or sleeping bag)? ☐ Yes ☐ No

34. If you answered yes, what happened?

_____

35. Have you ever been punished for wetting the bed? ☐ Yes ☐ No

36. If you answered yes, describe the punishment.

_____

_____

_____

37. Do your parents both agree about your doing the Waking Up Dry Program? ☐ Yes ☐ No

38. Is there any stress going on at home that may make it harder for your parents to work on the program with you? ☐ Yes ☐ No

39. If you answered yes, describe the problem.

_____

_____

40. Are your parents separated or divorced? ☐ Yes ☐ No

41. If you answered yes, how well do your parents communicate with each other?
    a. They communicate well about most issues.
    b. They communicate well if it involves their children.
    c. They don't communicate well about anything.

42. Is anyone in your family very sick or scheduled to have surgery in the next 2 months? ☐ Yes ☐ No

43. If you answered yes, describe what's happening.

    _____

    _____

44. Do you have brothers or sisters? ☐ Yes ☐ No

45. Is your brother or sister having any problems at home or school that might interfere with your working on the program? ☐ Yes ☐ No

46. If you answered yes, describe the problem.

    _____

    _____

    _____

47. Are you and your parents currently having problems such as arguing a lot about homework or family rules? ☐ Yes ☐ No

48. If you answered yes, what are the problems?

    _____

    _____

    _____

49. Are your parents planning to have or
adopt a baby in the next 2 months? ☐ Yes ☐ No

50. Are you planning to move or go on
vacation in the next 2 months? ☐ Yes ☐ No

51. Do your parents ask you not to drink
after dinner to help you stay dry? ☐ Yes ☐ No

52. If you answered yes, how much does this help?
   a. Not at all
   b. A little
   c. A lot

53. Have you tried anything in the past to
treat your bedwetting? ☐ Yes ☐ No

54. If you answered yes, write down what you did and whether
or not it helped.

_____

_____

_____

55. Were you ever dry at night for more than
6 months in a row? ☐ Yes ☐ No

56. How often do you wet the bed?
   a. Less than once per week
   b. One to 2 times per week
   c. Three to 4 times per week
   d. Five to 7 times per week

57. How many times do you wet the bed at night?
   a. Once
   b. Twice
   c. Three times
   d. Unsure

58. Do your parents have an idea of the times
    when you usually wet the bed? ☐ Yes ☐ No

59. If you answered yes, what times do you wet the bed?

    _____

60. When you wet the bed at night, do you go back to sleep
    in your own bed, or do you get in bed with someone else?

    _____

61. Have you ever wet someone else's bed
    after wetting your own? ☐ Yes ☐ No

62. If you answered yes, whose bed did you wet?

    _____

63. Do you ever wake up on your own to go
    to the bathroom? ☐ Yes ☐ No

64. If you answered yes, how often do you wake up?
    a. Occasionally
    b. Frequently
    c. Always

65. Are you a deep sleeper? ☐ Yes ☐ No

66. If you answered yes, how hard is it for your parents to wake
    you up?
    a. Not too hard
    b. Pretty hard
    c. Impossible

67. Do you ever wake up at night after you
    wet the bed? ☐ Yes ☐ No

68. If you answered yes, how often do you wake up?
    a. Occasionally
    b. Frequently
    c. Always

69. Do your parents take you to the bathroom
    after you go to sleep? ☐ Yes ☐ No

70. If you answered yes, how many times do they get you up?
    a. Once
    b. Twice
    c. Three times

71. If your parents take you to the bathroom, how often does
    this keep you dry?
    a. Always
    b. Sometimes
    c. Never

72. Are you dry if you sleep at a
    relative's house? ☐ Yes ☐ No

73. Do you wear Pull-Ups to bed? ☐ Yes ☐ No

74. If you answered yes, when do you wear them?
    a. All the time
    b. On special occasions, such as sleepovers and vacations
    c. If you are sick
    d. _____

75. Do you avoid going on sleepovers because
    you're wet at night? ☐ Yes ☐ No

76. If you go on sleepovers, how do you handle your
    bedwetting?
    a. Wear a Pull-Up.
    b. Tell your friend about the problem.
    c. Have someone take you to the bathroom in the middle of
       the night.
    d. _____

77. Do you take any responsibility for cleaning up in the morn-
    ing after having a wet bed? ☐ Yes ☐ No

78. If you answered yes, what responsibilities do you take?

_____

_____

_____

79. Do you pee during the day more than
    your friends?   ☐ Yes ☐ No

80. Does it seem like you often run to the
    bathroom at the last minute to pee?   ☐ Yes ☐ No

81. If you had to pee while you were riding in the car with
    your parents and you wouldn't be home for 15 minutes,
    what would you do?
    a. Hold back your urine with ease.
    b. Hold back your urine with difficulty.
    c. Ask your parents to pull over so you don't wet the seat.
    d. _____

82. How much do you want to be dry at night?
    a. A little
    b. A lot
    c. More than anything

83. What's the best thing that will happen when you become
    dry at night?

_____

_____

_____

_____

_____

_____

Extra Tips for Coaches

Because the bedwetting alarm wakes up children night after night, they can become tired and frustrated while they're doing the program. (Remember, it can take 3 to 4 months before a child becomes dry using the bedwetting alarm.) When I'm working with kids in my office, I have 2 jobs. My first job is to teach them how to become dry. My second job is to cheer them on. Although family members are as excited as I am when their kids start having dry nights, I like to call my patients on the phone to let them know I'm proud of them and pleased with how hard they're working. I can't take on this role for kids who are using the book, but you can step back from time to time and let your child know how proud you are of the efforts (and progress) he's making.

Things You Can Do During the Program

- Talk with your child once a week (until he's dry) to see how he's feeling about the program.
- Be supportive.
- Listen to your child (without criticism) if he feels like complaining about the program.
- Listen to your child (without criticism) if he feels like complaining that his progress is slower than he wants it to be.
- Tell your child what a good job he's doing.

- Don't push too hard if your child doesn't feel like talking about the program on any particular day.
- Remind your child that by practicing and sticking with the program, his chances of becoming dry get better and better.
- Check in with your child's doctor if you need additional help to make the program work.

Examples of Some Things You Can Say

- How is the program going?
- Is the program harder than you expected?
- I'm impressed with all the work you're doing to become dry at night.
- You sound tired. Are you irritated that the alarm woke you up last night?
- Should we call your doctor about any questions you have about becoming dry?
- Tell me what you're proud of so far.
- I remember when I was a kid, and I was learning how to _____. Some days went well, and others didn't. It frustrated me at the time, but now I realize that people always have ups and downs when they're learning something new.
- Are things going the way you hoped they would?
- What reward are you getting for this week's hard work?
- Does the program make it harder for you to be ready for school in the morning?
- Is there anything I can do to make the program work better?
- Is your brother or sister being helpful with the program? Is he or she being hurtful?
- Have any of your friends found out about the program?
- I'm so proud of you!
- I'm delighted you were dry last night!
- You're doing a great job!

- You're really good at remembering to do your exercises.
- What's the best thing that will happen when you're dry every night?

Think of some other things you can say and refer back to this section whenever you need to.

- _____

- _____

- _____

- _____

- _____

- _____

- _____

- _____

- _____

- _____

Tips for Medical Professionals

I stated in the introduction that one of my motivations for writing *Waking Up Dry* was to give children a program they could use at home with their parents. But I know from conversations with colleagues that the book can serve as a manual for health care professionals too. In truth, I hope most of the children who buy the book decide to use it with the support and encouragement of their doctors or nurse practitioners.

I also mentioned at the beginning of the book that practitioners might change some aspects of the program to fit their own approach to bedwetting. Nevertheless, I wrote this section to provide some additional information about the nuances of the program. I do not mean to be presumptuous, however, so please take the following information in the spirit in which it was intended.

How I Work With Children in the Office

I usually conduct my bedwetting consultations over two 30-minute visits. The first visit is informational. I make a tentative diagnosis, provide lots of details about the way the body works, and send the family home with instructions to evaluate the child's bowel and bladder habits. The second visit is treatment oriented. I assess the patient's motivation and build the program based on the child's individual needs.

Children are usually embarrassed or self-conscious at bed-wetting visits; therefore, I never start out asking them about their enuresis. I begin with a little small talk. Then I ask them lots of questions about their home, school, and hobbies. These questions not only let me ease into our bedwetting discussion but also provide valuable information about the child's world. For example, by watching how the child interacts with his parents, I get a sense of how well he communicates. By asking about the child's heroes, I learn about a person I can refer to later if he gets discouraged and I need to discuss what it takes to stick with the program. Asking questions about a child's home environment lets me know if there are any physical obstacles that may affect the program. For example, it's harder to use the enuresis alarm if a child's parents sleep on a different floor in the house.

My main goal at the first visit is to teach children how their bodies work and let them know why they're wet at night. I inform them that millions of kids wet the bed and there is nothing wrong with them. (Obviously, the specifics of this exchange are tailored to the child. If I have someone with daytime wetting or other problems, I alter what I say about his health.) I teach children how their nerves work, and we fill up balloons with water to see how the external sphincter muscle operates (sometimes they get wet by "accident"). I use a lot of repetition during the visit to make sure my patients understand what I'm teaching them, but I do so in an animated way and give them lots of positive feedback as we go along. If the child comes to the office with one parent, I ask him to "teach" the absent parent about the program that evening. I let him know that the parent who accompanied him to the office will help, but that he will be the one who does the teaching. This puts children in a position of authority, which they love.

When I give kids their dry-bed homework at the end of the first visit, I do it in a constructive manner. I often say something like, "Peter, you did a great job today. You really listened to what I had to say, and you learned a lot about your body. Remember that I'm the coach of the Waking Up Dry team and you're still trying out for the team. I have some homework for you to do so you can show me how much you want to be on the team. This homework is important because it gives me some information I need for the program and tells me if you're ready to become dry at night. However, from today's visit, I'm sure you are." At the end of the visit, I let the kids know that their parents will be my assistant coaches and they will help out with the homework. This approach works very well for children between the ages of 6 and 10 years. For older kids, I tone things down but communicate the same message.

If I sense some indifference on the child's part, I playact with him. Most of the time, I extend the sports example by pretending I'm the one who's trying out for the team. I act a little silly and use a whiny voice as I say things like, "Oh, man, I'm tired. I don't feel like practicing today." After a few moments, I ask the child how a coach would feel if a player behaved this way. I usually hear that the coach wouldn't like it. I then ask if a player is likely to make the team with this attitude. I usually hear that the player wouldn't make the team. I do all of this with an enthusiastic tone, guiding the child to the correct answers if necessary. By the end of the exchange, most kids are smiling and showing me the eagerness I like to see. I then tell them to go home and blast through their homework. I also remind them that they will be scoring goals in no time! (I adjust this comment based on the child's favorite sport or hobby.)

When kids come back for their second visit, I can tell fairly quickly how well I reeled them in at our first meeting. For example, if a child forgets his calendar or didn't do all of his homework, this usually means that he's not motivated enough to do the program. It's important to recognize, however, that kids have different temperaments, and quiet or introverted children may be more tentative during all phases of treatment.

The most important part of the second visit is determining if
the child is ready for the enuresis alarm (see Chapter 11). If a
child is not ready for the alarm, I suggest some simple behavioral measures to address the wetting. (In the book, I refer to
this as the Modified Waking Up Dry Program.) In many cases,
this is all that's needed to help a child become dry at night. If a
child is ready for the alarm, we set up the program at this visit.
This includes reviewing the various exercises the child will do
and going over the Waking Up Dry contract. Because I want
children to feel some degree of ownership for what we're doing,
I let them make some decisions about which elements we incorporate into the program.

I repeatedly emphasize that the child is the star of the show
but will also be the one does the most work. (This is a good time
to mention how much work his hero did to become a winner.)
I want children to realize that the more involved they are with
the program, the more likely it is they will succeed. A comment
I often make is, "Are you going to let your bladder be in charge
of you, or are you going to be in charge of your bladder?"

It's important to practice certain parts of the program in
the office so the child and parents can see the right way to do
things. This is especially true for waking up practice and the
enuresis alarm. I show kids some of the alarms described in
Chapter 17 (we review their pros and cons) and let them choose
the one they like best. Because it's impractical for you to buy
this many alarms, you can request brochures for these products
or keep a few models on hand to show patients.

I always rehearse the correct and incorrect way to respond
to a buzzing alarm. The first time I set off the alarm, the child
pretends to be so sleepy that he doesn't wake up. This gives
the parents a chance to practice the wake-up drill. The second
time I set off the alarm, the child wakes up quickly, turns off the

alarm, and pretends to pee in the bathroom. At the end of the visit, we review the program and I ask if there are any questions. I then tell the child that he's now part of the Waking Up Dry team. Even though it will take a lot of work, I remind him that his head coach and assistant coaches are here to help and, in time, he will become the boss of his body!

The most important thing to do at the beginning of the program is to give children positive feedback while they're still having lots of wet nights. To accomplish this, I call the family on a regular basis once the program begins. If a patient starts the program on a Friday night, I call the following Monday and weekly thereafter until steady progress is being made. I schedule additional office visits as needed but always want families to know I'm available to answer questions and fine-tune the program.

Although I avoid medication with most patients, there are a couple of circumstances in which the alarm itself may not be enough to help a child overcome his wetting: if a child is wetting multiple times per night or if a child is making very little progress 4 to 6 weeks into the program. Desmopressin is most likely to be effective in children with nocturnal polyuria who have a normal bladder capacity. Oxybutynin is most likely to be effective in children with a small bladder who set off their alarms multiple times per night.

Before I use medication with this group of patients, I have parents take them to the bathroom around 11:00 pm to try and reduce the number of wettings per night. If this doesn't work, I add a medication to the program. Once a child has been dry for 14 consecutive nights, I wean the lifting or medication over a 2- to 4-week period, adjusting my timing according to his clinical response.

The Waking Up Dry Program

Now that I've discussed my approach to bedwetting, let's review some rough numbers for the program. If a child passes the Alarm Clock Test, her chances of quitting are much lower than the 25% described in the literature; fewer than 10% of my patients drop out of treatment. My success rate for getting kids dry is also better than what is quoted in the literature (85% vs 50%–75%). The following 3 things contribute to this success:

• The program attacks bedwetting from different angles.

• I eliminate less motivated children before we start.

• I'm not dealing with a referral population, which may contain a higher percentage of children who are difficult to treat.

Approximately 15% of my patients relapse after becoming dry. Most of these patients become dry if they repeat the program.

Most children who quit the program do so because they aren't having the progress they hoped for or the program turned out to be harder than they expected. When this happens, I praise the child for her cooperation and comment on any aspect of the program that went well. I then ask if there is any part of the program that she would like to continue. If she says yes, I adjust the program accordingly, hoping to add other elements in the future. If the child isn't interested in continuing with the program, I tell her that's OK. The important thing is to minimize negative feelings about the program because that will make it more difficult for her to try again in the future.

Periodically, I see patients who tried really hard to become dry, but nothing worked or provided lasting results. When this happens, I tell the child I'm proud of the effort she made but that her body isn't cooperating with the program. I usually suggest that she take a break and try again in 6 to 12 months. In the interim, I recommend a scheduled lifting program, with 1 or 2 awakenings per night, to try and keep her dry. Another option in this situation is desmopressin. The *Physicians' Desk Reference* recommends using desmopressin for up to 6 months, though recent research suggests it's safe to use for longer periods.[1] If you prescribe desmopressin for more than 6 months, you should stop the medication every few months to see if the child still needs it. Finally, a small group of children require a combination of desmopressin and oxybutynin to attain nighttime dryness.[2]

I hope this information is useful and the book is a handy reference for teaching your patients to become dry at night.

References

1. Wolfish NM, Barkin J, Gorodzinsky F, Schwarz R. The Canadian Enuresis Study and Evaluation—short- and long-term safety and efficacy of an oral desmopressin preparation. *Scand J Urol Nephr.* 2003;37(1):22–27

2. Nevéus T. Oxybutynin, desmopressin and enuresis. *J Urol.* 2001;166(6):2459–2462

Supplemental Reading

Bedwetting Alarm

Bradbury M. Combination therapy for nocturnal enuresis with desmopressin and an alarm device. *Scandinavian Journal of Urology and Nephrology Supplement.* 1997;183:61–63

Butler RJ. Combination therapy for nocturnal enuresis. *Scandinavian Journal of Urology and Nephrology.* 2001;35(5):364–369

Butler RJ, Robinson JC. Alarm treatment for childhood nocturnal enuresis: an investigation of within-treatment variables. *Scandinavian Journal of Urology and Nephrology.* 2002;36(4):268–272

Hvistendahl GM, Kamperis K, Rawashdeh YF, Rittig S, Djurhuus JC. The effect of alarm treatment on the functional bladder capacity in children with monosymptomatic nocturnal enuresis. *Journal of Urology.* 2004;171(6):2611–2614

Kwak KW, Park KN, Baek M. The efficacy of enuresis alarm treatment in pharmacotherapy-resistant nocturnal enuresis. *Urology.* 2011;77(1):200–204

Bladder Mechanics

Butler RH. Exploring the differences between mono- and polysymptomatic nocturnal enuresis. *Scandinavian Journal of Urology and Nephrology.* 2006;40(4):313–319

De Wachter S, Vermandel A, De Moerloose K, Wyndaele JJ. Value of increase in bladder capacity in treatment of refractory monosymptomatic nocturnal enuresis in children. *Urology.* 2002;60(6):1090–1094

Kawauchi A, Tanaka Y, Naito Y, et al. Bladder capacity at the time of enuresis. *Urology.* 2003;61(5):1016–1018

Medication

Austin PF, Ferguson G, Yan Y. Combination therapy with desmopressin and an anticholinergic medication for non-responders to desmopressin for monosymptomatic nocturnal enuresis: a randomized, double-blind, placebo-controlled trial. *Pediatrics.* 2008;122(5):1027–1032

Butler RJ, Holland P, Robinson J. Examination of the structured withdrawal program to prevent relapse of nocturnal enuresis. *Journal of Urology.* 2001;166(6):2463–2466

Butler RJ, Robinson JC, Holland P, Doherty-Williams D. Investigating the three systems approach to complex childhood nocturnal enuresis—medical treatment interventions. *Scandinavian Journal of Urology and Nephrology.* 2004;38(2):117–121

Radvanska E, Kovacs L, Rittig S. The role of bladder capacity in antidiuretic and anticholinergic treatment for nocturnal enuresis. *Journal of Urology.* 2006;176(2):764–768

Robson WL, Norgaard JP, Leung AK. Hyponatremia in patients with nocturnal enuresis treated with DDAVP. *European Journal of Pediatrics.* 1996;155(11):959–962

Miscellaneous Topics

Austin PF, Ritchey ML. Dysfunctional voiding. *Pediatrics in Review.* 2000;21(10):336–341

Butler RJ, Heron J. The prevalence of infrequent bedwetting and nocturnal enuresis in childhood. *Scandanavian Journal of Urology and Nephrology.* 2008;42(3):257–264

Byrd RS, Weitzman M, Lamphear NE, et al. Bed-wetting in US children: epidemiology and related behavior problems. *Pediatrics.* 1996;98(3):414–419

Dunlop A. Meeting the needs of parents and pediatric patients: results of a survey on primary nocturnal enuresis. *Clinical Pediatrics.* 2005;44(4):297–303

El-Anany FG, Maghraby HA, Shaker SE, Abdel-Moneim AM. Primary nocturnal enuresis: a new approach to conditioning treatment. *Urology.* 1999;53(2):405–409

Honjo H, Kawauchi A, Ukimura O, Soh J, Mizutani Y, Miki T. Treatment of monosymptomatic nocturnal enuresis by acupuncture: a preliminary study. *International Journal of Urology.* 2002;9(12):672–676

Landgraf JM, Abidari J, Cilento BG, Cooper CS, Schulman SL, Ortenberg J. Coping, commitment, and attitude: quantifying the everyday burden of enuresis on children and their families. *Pediatrics.* 2004;113(2):334–344

Longstaffe S, Moffatt ME, Whalen JC. Behavioral and self-concept changes after six months of enuresis treatment: a randomized, controlled trial. *Pediatrics.* 2000;105(4):935–940

Nappo S, Del Gado R, Chiozza ML, Biraghi M, Ferrara P, Caione P. Nocturnal enuresis in the adolescent: a neglected problem. *BJU International.* 2002;90(9):912–917

O'Regan S, Yazbeck S, Hamberger B, Schick E. Constipation a commonly unrecognized cause of enuresis. *American Journal of Diseases of Children.* 1986;140(3):260–261

Robson WL. Diurnal enuresis. *Pediatrics in Review.* 1997;18(12): 407–412

Robson WL, Jackson HP, Blackhurst D, Leung AK. Enuresis in children with attention-deficit hyperactivity disorder. *Southern Medical Journal.* 1997;90(5):503–505

Van Kampen M, Bogaert G, Akinwuntan EA, Claessen L, Van Poppel H, De Weerdt W. Long-term efficacy and predictive factors of full spectrum therapy for nocturnal enuresis. *Journal of Urology.* 2004;171(6):2599–2602

von Gontard A, Schaumburg H, Hollman E, Eiberg H, Rittig S. The genetics of enuresis: a review. *Journal of Urology.* 2001;166(6):2438–2443

Review Articles

Caldwell PHY, Nankivell G. Sureshkumar P. Simple behavioural interventions for nocturnal enuresis in children. *The Cochrane Library.* 2013;7:1–19

Hjalmas K, Arnold T, Bower W, et al. Nocturnal enuresis: an international evidence based management strategy. *Journal of Urology.* 2004;171(6):2545–2561

Jalkut MW, Lerman SE, Churchill BM. Enuresis. *Pediatric Clinics of North America.* 2001;48(6):1461–1488

Lawless MR, McElderry DH. Nocturnal enuresis: current concepts. *Pediatrics in Review.* 2001;22(12):399–407

Robson WL. Evaluation and management of enuresis. *New England Journal of Medicine.* 2009;360(14):1429–1436

Schmitt BD. Nocturnal enuresis. *Pediatrics in Review.* 1997;18(6):183–191

Vandewalle J, Rittig S, Bauers S. Practical consensus guidelines for the management of enuresis. *European Journal of Pediatrics.* 2012;171(6):971–983

Sleep

Nevéus T. The role of sleep and arousal in nocturnal enuresis. *Acta Paediatrica.* 2003;92(10):1118–1123

Wolfish NM. Sleep/arousal and enuresis subtypes. *Journal of Urology.* 2001;166(6):2444–2447

Glossary

Alarm Clock Test. A method for determining if children can wake up at night, with or without their parents' help, in response to an alarm sound. If a child is able to wake up, he is a good candidate for the bedwetting alarm.

arousal disorder. A medical term used to describe people who are deep sleepers. Individuals with this condition have difficulty waking from sleep in response to internal or external stimuli (eg, sounds, touch, a full bladder).

bedwetting. See *enuresis*.

bedwetting alarm. A device that teaches children to become dry at night. The alarm consists of a wetness sensor that goes in a child's underpants and an alarm unit that buzzes, vibrates, or both when a child wets the bed at night.

bladder. A muscular pouch that stores urine until a person is ready to urinate.

bladder attention. One of the bladder exercises used in the Waking Up Dry Program. It teaches a child to be more aware of the signals her bladder sends prior to urination.

bladder capacity. The amount of urine the bladder can hold. Children who urinate frequently or feel a sense of urgency before they urinate often have a small functional bladder capacity.

constipation. The passage of large or hard stools. Constipation and infrequent defecation can cause daytime and nighttime wetting.

deep sleep. See *arousal disorder.*

defecation. The process of passing feces out of the body.

desmopressin. A manufactured form of vasopressin. Desmopressin treats bedwetting by reducing the amount of urine a child produces at night.

dry-bed homework. A series of tasks that children carry out to determine if they are motivated enough to work on becoming dry at night.

dysuria. A stinging or burning sensation that occurs during urination.

encopresis. Fecal soiling in a child older than 4 years. It is usually the result of stool withholding in a child with chronic constipation.

enuresis. The medical term for involuntary wetting in a child older than 5 years that is not caused by anatomic or neurologic disorders. If a child wets the bed at night, it is called *nocturnal enuresis.* If a child wets during the day, it is called *diurnal enuresis.* A child has *primary enuresis* if he never had 6 months of consistent dryness. A child has *secondary enuresis* if he had 6 months of consistent dryness and began wetting again.

enuresis alarm. The medical term for the bedwetting alarm.

fecal impaction. A large, hard plug of stool in the rectum. This can cause abdominal pain, fecal soiling, and enuresis.

feces. Solid waste that is eliminated from the intestinal tract.

frequency. The sensation of needing to urinate frequently.

hesitancy Difficulty starting urination. This can occur because of the pain associated with a urinary tract infection or because a child has a voiding dysfunction.

hormone. A chemical the body produces to regulate certain physiologic processes. Examples include thyroid hormone, growth hormone, and vasopressin.

hypnosis. A technique that uses visualization, imagery, and posthypnotic suggestions to help people lose weight or stop smoking. Hypnosis can also be used to help children become dry at night.

imipramine. A medication used by some doctors to treat bedwetting.

incontinence. Involuntary wetting that is caused by an anatomic abnormality or neurologic condition.

kidney. The organ responsible for eliminating excess water and certain waste products from the body.

laxative. A medication used to treat constipation. Laxatives stimulate the intestinal tract to work harder to push feces through the body.

lifting. The process of taking a child to the bathroom late in the evening to urinate. Parents typically do this before they go to bed themselves to prevent bedwetting episodes from occurring.

nocturnal polyuria. The medical term used to describe excessive urine production at night. This occurs in children who don't make enough vasopressin.

odor eliminators. Products that neutralize unpleasant odors.

overactive bladder. When a bladder fills with urine, it normally accommodates the increased volume without a sudden rise in pressure. An overactive bladder is unable to do this, which leads to uncontrolled bladder contractions and a sense of urgency and frequency in affected individuals.

overlearning. A technique used in conjunction with the bed-wetting alarm to reduce the chances that a child will relapse after a bedwetting program is complete.

oxybutynin. A medication that relaxes bladder muscles. It is usually given to relieve symptoms such as urgency, frequency, and daytime wetting.

pediatric nephrologist. A pediatrician that specializes in diseases of the kidney.

pediatric urologist. A pediatric surgeon that specializes in diseases of the urinary tract. Pediatric urologists are experts at managing bedwetting.

pelvic floor muscles. A group of muscles that supports the pelvic organs. The urethra and rectum pass through the pelvic floor.

Physicians' Desk Reference. A compendium of information on drugs and therapeutic agents used to treat medical disorders.

pituitary gland. This is the master gland of the body's endo-crine system. It is located at the base of the brain. (The *endo-crine system* is a collection of glands that control certain physiologic processes through the release of hormones.)

rectum. The last part of the large intestine. When feces collect in this area, a signal is sent to the brain alerting a person that it is time to defecate.

sphincter muscle. The muscle that encircles the urethra as it exits the bladder. This is the muscle a person squeezes to hold back urination or stop the urinary stream when voiding.

stool softener. A medication used to soften feces so they move through the intestinal tract more easily.

underpads. Disposable or reusable products that can be placed on a bed to protect the mattress from urine.

ureter. A small tube that drains urine from the kidney to the bladder.

urethra. The tube that carries urine from the bladder out of the body. In males, it passes through the pelvic floor into the penis. In females, it passes through the pelvic floor and terminates in an opening right above the vagina.

urgency. The sensation of needing to urinate very soon.

urinary tract. The system of organs responsible for the production and removal of urine from the body—kidney, ureter, bladder, and urethra.

urinary tract infection. A bacterial infection of the urinary tract. These infections can occur anywhere from the kidney to the bladder.

vasopressin. A hormone secreted by the pituitary gland that reduces the amount of urine produced at night. Some children wet the bed because they do not make enough of this hormone.

voiding. To void means "to empty." Doctors use the word voiding to describe the act of urinating.

voiding schedule. If a child has daytime wetting because of uncontrolled bladder contractions or because she doesn't feel her bladder signals, a timed voiding schedule will often keep her dry. This involves going to the bathroom at regular intervals, usually every 2 hours.

wake-up drill. A technique used to help children wake up in response to the bedwetting alarm.

Waking Up Dry calendar. The record children use to track their progress as they do the Waking Up Dry Program.

Waking Up Dry contract. The contract children and coaches sign at the beginning of the Waking Up Dry Program. It ensures that everyone knows what is expected during the program.

waking up practice. One of the behavioral components of the Waking Up Dry Program. Before children go to sleep at night, they lie in bed and practice getting up to go to the bathroom. This teaches them to go to the bathroom if they need to urinate during the night.

water gulping. One of the bladder exercises used in the Waking Up Dry Program. By drinking more during the day, children get more practice going to the bathroom. This regulates their voiding pattern and makes it more likely they will respond to their bladders at night.

Index

Page numbers in *italic* denote figures and tables.

Z

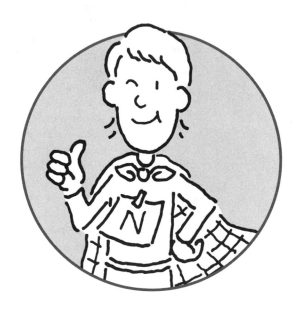